Cocaine

Roger D. Weiss, M.D.
and
Steven M. Mirin, M.D.

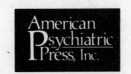

1400 K Street, N.W.
Washington, DC 20005

Note: The authors have worked to ensure that all information in this book concerning drug dosages, schedules, and routes of administration is accurate at the time of publication and consistent with standards set by the United States Food and Drug Administration and the general medical community. As medical research and practice advance, however, therapeutic standards may change. For this reason, and because human and mechanical errors sometimes occur, we recommend that readers follow the advice of a physician directly involved in their care or the care of a member of their family.

Books published by the American Psychiatric Press, Inc., represent the views and opinions of the individual authors and do not necessarily reflect the policies and opinions of the Press or the American Psychiatric Association.

Cover design by Tom Engeman
Text design by Richard E. Farkas
Typeset by Unicorn Graphics
Printed by RR Donnelley & Sons Co.

First Printing

Library of Congress Cataloging-in-Publication Data

Weiss, Roger D., 1951–
   Cocaine.

   Bibliography: p.
   Includes index.
   1. Cocaine habit.   2. Cocaine—Physiological
effect.   3. Cocaine habit—United States.   4. Cocaine habit—
Treatment.   I. Mirin, Steven M., 1942–   . II. Title.
[DNLM: 1. Cocaine. 2. Substance Abuse.   WM 280 W432c]
RC568.C6W46   1987   616.86′3   86-17245
ISBN 0-88048-216-8 (alk. paper)

*To our families, in appreciation
of their understanding and support.*

Contents

About the Authors   xi
Preface   xiii

1. **The Current Cocaine Epidemic**   1
   The Scope of the Problem   1
   Cocaine Use Through History   4
   From Coca Leaf to the American Street   8

2. **How Cocaine Is Used**   13
   Intranasal Cocaine Use ("Snorting")   13
   Smoking Cocaine   16
   Intravenous Cocaine Use   21

3. **The Effects of Cocaine on the Body**   23
   The General Physical Effects of Cocaine   24
   Medical Complications from Cocaine   25
   Cocaine Overdose   27
   How Cocaine Can Kill   27
   Effects of Long-Term Cocaine Use   29
   Medical Complications Due to Effects of Cocaine
      Itself   29
   Medical Complications Due to Drug
      Paraphernalia   32
   Medical Complications Due to Adulterants
      ("Cuts")   37
   Medical Complications Due to Life-Style and
      Psychiatric Symptoms in Cocaine Abusers   38

4. **Cocaine and the Brain** 41
    Basic Elements of Brain Function: The Nerve
      Cell   41
    Events at the Nerve Cell Junction (Synapse)   42
    The Effects of Cocaine on Brain Function   45
    Behavioral Effects of Long-Term Cocaine
      Use   49
    Adverse Reactions to Cocaine: Who Is
      Vulnerable?   53

5. **Cocaine Dependence** 55
    Factors Contributing to Cocaine Dependence   57
    The Course of Cocaine Dependence   73
    How Dependence Develops   74
    One Cocaine Addict's Story: Ellen   80

6. **Cocaine and the Family** 91
    Family Responses to the Cocaine Abuser   93
    How Families Try to Avoid the Pain of
      Cocaine Dependence   95
    How Relatives Can Help   101
    Recovery for the Families of Cocaine
      Abusers   103

7. **Cocaine in the Workplace** 107
    Why Cocaine?   108
    Hazards of Cocaine Use in the Workplace   109
    Cocaine Use by Executives   111
    The Response of Business   114
    The Concept of Employee Assistance   116

8. **Treatment of Cocaine Abuse** 121
    Getting the Cocaine Abuser into Treatment   122
    Treatment Methods for Cocaine Abusers   124
    How to Choose the Right Type of Treatment   135
    Seven General Rules for Cocaine Abusers Who Want
      to Quit   136
    Pathways to Recovery   139

9. **Questions Frequently Asked About Cocaine**   141
   Questions Frequently Asked by the General
     Public   141
   Questions Frequently Asked by Occasional
     Cocaine Users   142
   Questions Frequently Asked by People Dependent
     upon Cocaine   146
   Questions Frequently Asked by Those Who Treat
     Cocaine Abusers   150
   Questions Frequently Asked by Family
     Members of Cocaine Abusers   152

   Appendix A: Self-Test for Cocaine
     Dependence   155
   Appendix B: Where to Find Help: A State-by-State
     Guide to Cocaine Abuse Treatment
     Facilities   159
   Appendix C: Bibliography   169

   Index   175

About the Authors

Drs. Weiss and Mirin are psychiatrists who have worked together for nearly a decade in the treatment and study of drug-dependent individuals. Dr. Weiss is currently Director of the Alcohol and Drug Abuse Treatment Center at McLean Hospital in Belmont, Massachusetts. Dr. Mirin is the Medical Director of Westwood Lodge Hospital in Westwood, Massachusetts, and a Research Psychiatrist at the Alcohol and Drug Abuse Research Center of McLean Hospital, Belmont, Massachusetts.

Both authors are members of the faculty of Harvard Medical School, where Dr. Weiss is Assistant Professor of Psychiatry and Dr. Mirin is Associate Clinical Professor of Psychiatry. Each has lectured widely and contributed numerous articles to the medical and scientific literature on the abuse of cocaine and other drugs.

Preface

In recent years, cocaine use in the United States has reached epidemic proportions. A 1982 survey by the National Institute on Drug Abuse reported that 22 million Americans had used cocaine at least once, and medical complications and deaths from the drug over the last decade have each risen approximately 10-fold. The popularity of cocaine has spawned and supported a huge illegal network dedicated to its manufacture, importation, and distribution. The cost of cocaine use to industry in lost productivity, job-related accidents, claims for health care benefits, and poor employee morale may be more than 10 billion dollars a year. The personal cost to cocaine abusers, their families, and their friends is incalculable.

Although much has been written about various aspects of cocaine abuse, we felt that there was a need for a comprehensive overview of the problem. We have written *Cocaine* in order to provide that overview. This book is for those whose lives have been, or may be, affected by cocaine, and for those who work with cocaine abusers. We will discuss what cocaine is, the different methods of use, its effects on the brain and other organs, and its psychological and social consequences for users and those around them, both at home and in the workplace. We will also discuss cocaine dependence (addiction)—how it happens, who is at risk, how to treat it, and how to find help. *Cocaine* includes a list of commonly asked questions about cocaine, a self-test for cocaine dependence, and a nationwide list of cocaine abuse treatment facilities.

Much of what we have learned about cocaine abuse has been gained through our experience working with patients on the Drug Dependence Treatment Unit at McLean Hospital in Belmont, Massachusetts. We are grateful to the staff who have worked so hard to make that program successful and to the patients who have shared their experiences with us. In relating those experiences here, we have changed their names and other details about their lives in order to protect their anonymity.

Finally, we are grateful to Evelyn Stone for her encouragement and suggestions about the manuscript; Tim Clancy of the American Psychiatric Press for his support and helpful advice; Charles Weingarten, Scott Lukas, Eric Dessain, and Jacqueline Michael, all of whom reviewed sections of the book and contributed helpful comments; and Marjorie Maxwell and Jeanette Austin, who worked tirelessly and enthusiastically on the manuscript through its many revisions. We are also most grateful to The Charles Engelhard Foundation for its long-standing support of the clinical research component of our program.

Roger D. Weiss, M.D.
Steven M. Mirin, M.D.

1

The Current Cocaine Epidemic

The Scope of the Problem

No drug has attained as much popularity, notoriety, and controversy during the past decade as cocaine. Once a relatively obscure pastime of jazz musicians and film stars, the use of cocaine has recently become the subject of national magazine cover stories, movies, television shows, songs, and books. Although evidence citing the hazards of cocaine is steadily mounting, the number of people who use the drug continues to grow. For example, a 1974 survey conducted by the National Institute on Drug Abuse revealed that approximately five million Americans had used cocaine at least once. By 1982, that figure had reached 22 million. In 1973, less than 1 percent of university students responding to a survey on drug use admitted to having tried cocaine. Nine years later, in a similar study, 30 percent of the student population had used the drug. Unfortunately, the use of cocaine in America is not confined to adults: a 1985 national survey revealed that 17 percent of American high school seniors had tried cocaine; over one-third of that group had used the drug within the previous month.

The rising population of cocaine users has been accompanied by a similar increase in the number of heavy abusers who have had to seek medical treatment because of cocaine-related difficulties. For example, the number of medical emergencies due to cocaine increased by 900 percent between 1976 and 1985, while cocaine-related deaths increased by over 1100 percent. During this period, the percentage of cocaine-related admissions to drug abuse treatment facilities rose from 1.2 percent in 1976 to 9 percent in 1983. This represents a 750 percent increase over a seven-year period.

One result of the increasing popularity of cocaine has been a burgeoning international underground industry dedicated to the manufacture and distribution of the drug. Because of the great success of this business, cocaine is now readily available in most areas of the United States. As the supply of cocaine has grown, its market value, or price, has fallen. In the past several years, the cost of cocaine has declined from $150 a gram to approximately half that in many urban centers. This decline has reduced one of the major barriers to cocaine use for many individuals: its expense. The lowered cost has made it easier for some people to experiment with cocaine; it has been estimated that, every day, 5000 people use cocaine for the first time. Although some of those individuals may never try it again, others continue to use cocaine, and some eventually develop severe problems because of the drug.

One consequence of the growing availability and declining cost of cocaine has been the "democratization" of the drug. In the mid-1970s, "the champagne of drugs" was depicted primarily as part of the exclusive world of the rich and glamorous. Celebrities touted the drug's ability to induce stimulation safely; rock musicians saluted cocaine in their lyrics; stories in magazines and newspaper gossip columns described Hollywood parties at which film stars served cocaine to their guests in crystal bowls.

Today, however, cocaine is no longer exclusively a drug for the affluent. In fact, a 1984 study by E. D. Wish found that 69 percent of individuals arrested for drug-related offenses in East Harlem had traces of cocaine in their urine, while only half of the urine samples obtained were positive for opiate (narcotic) drugs such as heroin or methadone. Moreover, nearly half of the arrested group stated that they were dependent on cocaine—nearly twice the number of individuals who admitted to being addicted to heroin. Cocaine has become a widely prevalent drug that is being used at all levels of our society by men and women, adolescents and adults, rich and poor.

Accompanying the increasing population of cocaine users has been a growing trend toward increasingly dangerous patterns of cocaine abuse. Among patients visiting emergency rooms in 1982 for cocaine-related complications, 71 percent were also using other drugs, as opposed to 57 percent in 1978. Approximately one-quarter of these emergency-room patients were using cocaine in combination with heroin, a potentially deadly practice known as "speedballing." Another particularly disturbing trend is the shift among many cocaine users from intranasal use (snorting) to intravenous use and, more recently, to cocaine freebase smoking (freebasing). The use of freebase or intravenous cocaine is even more hazardous than intranasal use, because of the increased number of attendant medical complications and the higher likelihood of addiction associated with these methods of cocaine use. A 1982 survey of cocaine-related hospitalizations revealed a sevenfold increase in the number of admissions for freebasing, when compared with a similar study performed only three years previously.

The rise in freebase smoking appears likely to continue because of the recent introduction of "crack" (also known as "rock") into the drug marketplace. Crack is prepackaged cocaine freebase, which is available in small quantities ($10–$15) and sold ready to smoke. Some scientists consider crack the most addicting drug currently available on the street. Since its low initial price and easy use make crack especially appealing to adolescents, we may be on the verge of an epidemic of teenage cocaine addiction.

What is the appeal of cocaine? What does it do for people? How do people get enticed by this drug and then caught in its grip? What does it do to the mind? The body? The bankbook? The family? How does it affect people's jobs? How can people stop using it once they've started? What can a person do if a family member or friend is using cocaine? These are some of the issues that we will address in this book. In order to gain some perspective on the current cocaine epidemic, however, let us begin by looking at cocaine's place in history.

Cocaine Use Through History

Cocaine is a naturally occurring stimulant drug found in the leaves of the coca plant, *Erythroxylon coca*. Although cocaine was not extracted from the coca leaf until the mid-19th century, archeologists have discovered coca leaves at Peruvian gravesites from approximately 500 A.D., along with other items considered necessities for the afterlife. Thus, although current practices of cocaine use are relatively recent by historical standards, coca leaves have been chewed for at least 15 centuries.

Coca leaves have been used in the past for a variety of religious, medicinal, and work-related reasons. They have also been the subject of a great deal of folklore over the years. Many inhabitants of coca-growing regions believed that the leaf was of divine origin, and its use was therefore reserved for members of the upper classes. One Incan myth described coca as an herb provided by the god Inti to allow the Incas to endure their difficult environmental conditions without suffering from hunger or thirst. Another myth alleged that the coca plant grew from the remains of a beautiful woman who had been executed for adultery, cut in half, and buried. Themes of seductiveness and danger have thus been associated with cocaine for well over a millennium.

After conquering the Incas in the 16th century, the Spanish were initially opposed to coca use because they saw worship of the drug as a barrier to religious conversion. However, the conquistadores also recognized that the leaves energized the Indians and enabled them to work long, tedious hours in gold and silver mines with little need for food or sleep. Financial considerations overcame their religious objections, and in 1569, Phillip II of Spain declared the coca habit essential to the health of the Indian. It was not long thereafter that the Spaniards began paying the Indians with coca leaves. Around this time, coca also developed a reputation as being able to treat a variety of medical disorders, including such diverse conditions as venereal diseases, headaches, asthma, rheumatism, and toothaches.

Despite the imprimatur of the Spaniards who brought coca leaves back to Europe, there was very little enthusiasm among the Europeans for coca until 1855, when a German chemist named Friedrich Gaedecke was able to extract the active ingredient of the coca leaf, which he named *erythroxyline*. In 1859, fellow countryman Albert Niemann also isolated the compound, which he renamed *cocaine*. This discovery sparked a flourish of experimentation with the compound, which peaked around the turn of the century. Perhaps the most notable of the drug's champions was Sigmund Freud, who performed a great deal of research on the drug, based both on personal experience and on the observation of others. In July 1884, Freud published his landmark paper, entitled "On Coca." In this work, he rhapsodized about the effects of cocaine as follows:

> The psychic effect of cocaine consists of exhilaration and lasting euphoria, which does not differ in any way from the normal euphoria of a healthy person. . . . One senses an increase of self-control and feels more vigorous and more capable of work; on the other hand, if one works, one misses the heightening of the mental powers which alcohol, tea, or coffee induces. One is simply normal, and soon finds it difficult to believe that one is under the influence of any drug at all. . . . Long lasting intensive mental or physical work can be performed without fatigue; it is as though the need for food and sleep, which otherwise makes itself felt peremptorily at certain times of the day, were completely banished.

Freud also noted the drug's ability to relieve pain, and thus paved the way for the discovery of cocaine as the first local anesthetic. He also claimed that cocaine might prove useful as a stimulant, as an aphrodisiac, and in the treatment of depression, gastrointestinal disturbances, wasting diseases, alcoholism, morphine addiction, and asthma. None of these predictions was supported by scientific research, and Freud was accused of irresponsibility by much of the scientific community because of his enthusiasm for cocaine. When Freud used the drug in order to treat a colleague for morphine addiction, he was dismayed to find his patient develop a similar severe dependence on cocaine. This and other developments led Freud to eventually modify his positive feelings about cocaine.

Sigmund Freud was not the only person in the late 19th century to embrace this new compound. A Corsican chemist named Angelo Mariani understood the power of this newly discovered drug, and he realized that there was money to be made from cocaine. Thus in 1863, Mariani produced a mixture of coca leaves and wine, which he called Vin Mariani. This tonic was phenomenally successful: among those who endorsed it were kings, queens, two popes, and such notable figures as Thomas Edison, H. G. Wells, and Jules Verne.

In 1886, an American chemist named John Styth Pemberton created a new patent medicine that was advertised as "a valuable Brain tonic and cure for all nervous affections—SICK HEADACHE, NEURALGIA, HYSTERIA, MELANCHOLY, etc." This patent medicine was later promoted as a soft drink with cocaine as its major active ingredient. Thus, Coca Cola was born. Americans as well as Europeans were thus discovering around the turn of the century what South American Indians had known for hundreds of years: that the coca leaf could energize them, lift them up, and make them feel good. Although caffeine has since been substituted for cocaine as the active ingredient in Coca Cola, decocainized coca leaves are still included as part of the beverage's "natural flavors."

Cocaine use was also popularized in turn-of-the-century literature; no less a figure than Sherlock Holmes injected the drug regularly. Eventually, however, in the early part of the 20th century, this unrestrained enthusiasm for cocaine began to be tempered by increasing evidence of the drug's addictive properties. In addition, broader social factors coincided to dampen this fascination with cocaine. For example, certain "muckraking" journalists began to attack manufacturers of patent medicines because the reporters felt that the outlandish claims made for these tonics represented attempts to dupe the general public. This effort was joined by American physicians, who were becoming an increasingly organized and professional group. In addition, popular newspapers wrote about the relationship between cocaine and criminal behavior. This movement, which took a decidedly racist tone, resulted in reports of murders by "crazed (black) cocaine takers" and "attacks upon white women of the South ... [as] the direct result of [the] coke-crazed negro brain."

This combination of events led to restrictions on cocaine under the Federal Harrison Narcotics Act of 1914. The Act was a paradoxical piece of legislation because it incorrectly classified cocaine as a narcotic, when in fact the drug is a stimulant. In addition, 46 of the 48 states at that time passed similar legislation to curb cocaine use, whereas only 29 states had similar laws concerning true narcotic drugs. From 1914 until the early 1970s, cocaine use "went underground." Use was largely confined to the fast and loose—movie stars, jazz musicians, and wealthy thrill seekers. However, it was not used frequently by other members of the general public. Its illegal status made its price tag quite high, and a reasonable substitute in the form of amphetamine was available cheaply and legally, by prescription.

It is difficult to explain the overwhelming resurgence of cocaine use in this country beginning in the early 1970s. A number of factors, however, converged to change the drug-taking habits of America. First, an increasing segment of America had grown up using drugs. The use of marijuana and hallucinogens in the 1960s by a significant number of young Americans made many of them unafraid of the legal and potential medical consequences of so-called "soft" drug use. Unfortunately, cocaine had developed a reputation as being a "soft" and "safe" drug: nonaddicting, not dangerous, short-acting—the perfect social drug. It became the drug of the rich and the powerful. Rock musicians sang its praises. Popular films portrayed cocaine as a glamorous, harmless plaything. Newspapers publicized arrests of film stars and sports celebrities who were apprehended for possession of the drug. Cocaine developed a mystique around it. Amphetamine, meanwhile, had acquired a bad reputation in the 1960s; the phrase "speed kills" had become well known among members of the drug culture. Prescriptions for amphetamine became increasingly regulated. There was thus a segment of American society that was looking for a new stimulant drug.

At the same time, new government efforts were being made to restrict the importation of marijuana from Mexico and opiates from the Far East. Since drug dealers are quite resourceful and are far more committed to staying in business than to any single drug, some of the business that was being impeded by law enforcement efforts was diverted and focused on the cocaine trade.

The substitution of cocaine for amphetamine as the stimulant of choice in America is a rather interesting one, because a study by a group of researchers from the University of Chicago found that experienced cocaine users were unable to distinguish between the effects of cocaine and amphetamine when alternately administered both drugs intravenously without being told which was which. Other experiments have shown that cocaine abusers have difficulty distinguishing between cocaine and intravenous lidocaine (Xylocaine) under similar conditions. What then, are cocaine abusers paying for? It appears to be more than just the pharmacological effect of the drug. Cocaine use offers a sense of power and prestige that is not present with any other drug. However, this is an illusory experience, since even people with power and prestige can easily lose control of their lives as the result of this powerful and humbling drug.

From Coca Leaf to the American Street

The manufacture and distribution of illicit cocaine is big business. In 1984, while marijuana and opium production levels were declining, the production of cocaine increased by approximately 30 percent. In order to meet the rising consumer demand in the United States, Europe, and South America, the farmers growing coca leaves and the drug smugglers, processors, and traffickers have had to devise increasingly ingenious and effective methods to keep pace. As law enforcement efforts have increased, the response of cocaine kingpins has become more sophisticated and, when necessary, more menacing and sanguinary.

The Manufacture of Cocaine

The conversion of the coca leaf to the product that is illicitly marketed on the American street as "cocaine" (the quotation marks are included because the product sold on the street often contains more adulterants than pure drug) involves many steps. It begins with the coca plant itself, *Erythroxylon coca,* an evergreen shrub approximately three feet tall that grows most commonly in the eastern foothills of the Andes Mountains. Over two hundred strains of coca plants have been identified. Although all contain some active alkaloids, the vast majority contain little if any cocaine. The bush thrives at elevations ranging between 1500 and 5000 feet and generally contains a relatively small amount of active cocaine; the average Peruvian coca leaf contains approximately one-half of one percent cocaine. The bitter taste of the alkaloids probably contributes to the flourishing growth of the coca bush by making the visually attractive bush an uninviting grazing source for the local animal population.

The coca plant can be harvested between six months and three years after its first planting, depending on the strain that has been planted. Once a growing area has been established, the leaves can be harvested several times a year, simply by stripping the leaves off the bushes. The farmers then take the harvested leaves to local processing plants located in the villages, where the initial stage of extraction takes place. Here, coca paste is prepared by macerating coca leaves with kerosene, water, sodium carbonate, and sulfuric acid. Between 100 and 200 kilograms of coca leaves are necessary to produce one kilogram (2.2 pounds) of coca paste. The conversion of the leaf to paste thus results in an enormous reduction in bulk as well as an increasingly (40–91 percent) pure product now worth four times the price of the original leaves. The decreased bulk enables drug traffickers to transport coca paste far more easily than they can move massive quantities of coca leaves. Coca paste is converted into cocaine hydrochloride, the snowy white powder sold on the American street, by adding a number of chemicals, which may include hydrochloric acid, potassium permanganate, acetone, ether, ammonia, calcium carbonate, sodium carbonate, sulfuric acid, and more kerosene.

Meanwhile, the price of the product has been steadily escalating. It takes approximately 2.5 kilograms of coca paste to produce a kilogram of pure cocaine hydrochloride, with a concomitant tripling of the price. In addition, the smuggling of cocaine from South America to the United States is a risky business; participants therefore expect to be well compensated for their efforts. Thus, the price of cocaine is again increased by approximately 300 percent after it has been illegally exported to the United States. Unfortunately, the manufacture of cocaine for street distribution does not end with the smuggling of cocaine into the United States. Rather, the drug is then distributed from large drug traffickers to a series of increasingly smaller drug dealers. In each of these transactions, adulterants are added to the cocaine in order to make it less pure and thus more profitable to sell. As cocaine usage has become increasingly popular, the purity of the drug sold on the streets has fluctuated. In 1976, street samples submitted to drug analysis laboratories averaged 53–73 percent cocaine. Although estimates of cocaine purity in the early 1980s were considerably lower, averaging between 20 and 40 percent, recent reports have cited an increase in the purity of street cocaine—an ominous trend for addiction potential when combined with lower prices. If we conservatively estimate the purity of a street sample of cocaine to be 25 percent, the price will have quadrupled again between importation into the United States and distribution to the user. The net price increase, then, from coca leaf to the purchase of cocaine on the street is approximately 15,000 percent. The current price of cocaine on the American street ranges from $50–$100 for a gram (1/28th of an ounce).

The Uphill Battle Against the Cocaine Trade

Illicit drug trafficking is conservatively estimated to be a 100 billion dollar a year business. Despite numerous efforts by the United States government to halt the overwhelming flow of cocaine into this country, production of the coca leaf increased by 30 percent in 1984; in Bolivia, production has tripled in the last seven years. New countries such as Venezuela, Paraguay, and Trinidad, heretofore uninvolved in the drug trade, have recently entered the coca business because of its steady growth and enormous profitability.

The history of attempts to curb the cocaine trade has been marked by great frustration. For example, as law enforcement efforts have focused on eradication of local refineries in Bolivia and Peru, similar operations have been begun in Venezuela, Panama, and Argentina. When federal drug enforcement agents began to impede drug traffic coming into Miami, traditionally the chief American port for cocaine, new smuggling routes emerged, with ports of entry in Texas, Arizona, California, and Mexico. Coca bushes and cocaine refineries have even been found recently in the United States.

When law enforcement agencies have focused less on drug smuggling and more on the coca plants themselves, efforts have been similarly difficult. For example, attempts to eradicate the coca leaf in Peru and Bolivia have resulted in a flourishing coca crop in Ecuador and Brazil. The difficulty of this strategy was dramatically illustrated when a group of Peruvian workers who had been paid by the United States to uproot and burn coca bushes were tortured and murdered. In some countries, such as Bolivia, growing and selling coca leaves is perfectly legal; natives drink coca leaf tea like Americans drink coffee or Coca Cola, for an energizing lift. The United States government has sponsored programs to encourage South American nations to grow other crops such as coffee instead of coca leaves. However, it is very difficult to convince subsistence farmers and poor nations to cease growing their only profitable crop. Indeed, there have been efforts in some countries to grow coca more efficiently. In the Amazon River basin of Brazil, for example, a new strain of coca bush known as epadu is being cultivated. Epadu, unlike *Erythroxylon coca,* can flourish in the jungle and can grow to a height of 10 feet.

The efforts of the United States government to stop the cocaine trade are therefore being thwarted because law enforcement officials are caught between two very powerful forces: American cocaine users, who desperately want the drug, and drug manufacturers and traffickers, who are equally motivated to sell their product. When the pressure is placed at the source, i.e., at those growing and refining coca leaves, they respond by cultivating a heartier plant, moving their operations elsewhere, and threatening law enforcement agents. When the law exerts pressure further down the line, the resultant capture and destruction of large cocaine shipments into the United States results in a Pyrrhic victory: an increase in the street price of cocaine. While this may discourage some potential users, it will lead to increased illegal activity among those who will use the drug at any price. As one hospitalized cocaine abuser said after reading of a large-scale cocaine bust, "It looks like the price of cocaine just went up today. If I were still out on the street, I guess I'd have to come up with another sleazy way to get even more money that I don't have."

2

How Cocaine Is Used

Intranasal Cocaine Use ("Snorting")

The most common method of cocaine use in the United States today is intranasal use, or "snorting." A recent survey by Dr. Mark Gold and his coworkers at the 1-800-COCAINE telephone helpline revealed that 61 percent of the callers to their center used the drug intranasally. Users prepare crystalline cocaine hydrochloride purchased on the street by placing it on a flat shiny surface—typically, a mirror, a glass coffee table, or a piece of marble. The cocaine is then chopped finely with a razor blade and arranged into thin lines approximately an eighth of an inch wide and one or two inches long. Approximately 30 to 40 lines can be made from one gram of cocaine, which is purchased on the street for $50 to $100. A line of cocaine is inhaled, often with great ceremony, through a straw, a rolled-up dollar bill or a thin cylindrical object called a "tooter." Although they are often made of glass, tooters made from valuable metals such as gold or even platinum are purchased by some drug users as a status symbol.

The amount of active drug present in a line of cocaine varies, depending upon the amount of adulterant that has been added. If the drug is only 10 percent pure, one line will contain only about 3 milligrams of pure cocaine. If, on the other hand, the cocaine is 50 percent pure, a line may contain approximately

15 milligrams of active drug. These figures assume importance because research has shown that volunteers given less than 10 milligrams of pure cocaine intranasally are unable to distinguish the effects of the drug from a placebo. Since street cocaine is sometimes so impure that a line may contain less than 10 milligrams of active drug, the pharmacological effect from such a preparation should be negligible. However, many drug users continue to get "high" from an amount of drug which has been shown in scientific experiments to be no more powerful than an inactive white powder. Thus, there must be more factors involved in the experience of cocaine intoxication than the direct chemical effect of the drug.

It is a well-known phenomenon among researchers and drug users that a person's experience while on a drug is strongly affected by the setting in which he uses the drug and the expectations he has of the drug's effects. For example, if someone anticipates becoming intoxicated, he is more likely to feel "high" after using a drug than is someone who expects to feel nothing. Getting high is thus, in part, a learned experience: one learns how to act, how to feel, and what sensations to anticipate and guard against. This phenomenon was illustrated clearly in a fascinating study of marijuana smokers by Dr. Reese Jones at the University of California, San Francisco. In this study, many individuals who unknowingly smoked marijuana cigarettes with little or no tetrahydrocannabinol (THC, the psychoactive ingredient in marijuana) claimed to feel intoxicated when they thought they were smoking bona fide marijuana.

We have discussed these phenomena in order to underscore the importance of nonpharmacological factors involved in the cocaine experience—the importance of rituals, crisp new hundred dollar bills through which some people inhale cocaine, solid gold tooters and "coke spoons" for snorting, and special "cutting kits." These consist of little more than a few razor blades, mirrors, and straws, but can cost $20 or more.

Effects of Intranasal Use

After inhalation, cocaine is rapidly absorbed into the bloodstream—first into the small blood vessels of the nose, and then into the general circulation. The drug can be detected in the blood within three minutes after use, and the amount of drug present in the blood (the *blood level*) increases quickly, peaking between 15 minutes and an hour after the drug has been taken.

The effects of cocaine on mood are most prominent 15 to 30 minutes after intranasal administration. Cardiovascular changes, including an increased heart rate and blood pressure, occur most strongly in 15 to 20 minutes. Although the emotional and cardiovascular effects of cocaine wear off approximately an hour after intranasal use, the drug remains in the bloodstream for four to six hours. One reason that cocaine may remain in the body so long is its ability to constrict the blood vessels in the nose, thus retarding the absorption of the drug into the general circulation. Indeed, cocaine can be detected in the nose for up to three hours after drug use. The discrepancy between the drug's brief duration of action and its prolonged presence in the blood may also be explained by the theory that cocaine makes people euphoric only as the amount of drug in the blood is rising. When the blood level plateaus and decreases, the drug may have little effect. In some cases, users with falling blood levels may feel as if they are coming off of the drug.

Although some people who use cocaine experience few untoward effects after occasional use, other individuals feel anxious, depressed, tired, and irritable approximately an hour after snorting small amounts of the drug. These symptoms may be accompanied by a desire for more cocaine. Although it is not known how many people in the general population have the latter response to cocaine use, a study by Dr. Richard Resnick and his colleagues at New York Medical College found that a subgroup of experienced cocaine users who volunteered for a study on the effects of cocaine experienced this "crash" or "post-coke blues" after taking 25 milligrams (approximately two lines) of cocaine intranasally. In these and other vulnerable individuals, a combination of post-cocaine depression, drug craving, and drug availability may lead to repetitive use, and—in some cases—cocaine dependence.

Medical Complications of Intranasal Use

Physical symptoms frequently experienced by intranasal cocaine users include nasal congestion and cold symptoms; in severe cases, they may suffer from ulceration of nasal tissue and, less often, perforation of the nasal septum (the hard portion of the nose between the two nostrils). Some individuals attempt to avert these difficulties by cleaning their noses with a saltwater solution or by using glycerine, vitamin E, or petroleum jelly (Vaseline). These home remedies and prophylactic measures are generally unsuccessful if cocaine use continues. Frequent use of nasal decongestants, particularly nasal sprays, is also common among intranasal cocaine users. Some individuals can become dependent upon these sprays and may experience a worsening of their symptoms when they try to discontinue these over-the-counter preparations. Specialized medical treatment may be necessary in order to wean such individuals from their nasal sprays.

Because intranasal administration is by far the most common form of cocaine use, the patterns of use among this group vary widely. Whereas intravenous injection of cocaine generally implies heavy involvement with the drug, intranasal use may be seen in those who try the drug once out of curiosity, as well as in addicts who spend thousands of dollars a week on the drug. Many people have gathered the impression that "only snorting" cocaine is safe, and that it is very difficult to become addicted to cocaine via this "harmless" route of administration. Unfortunately, this idea has been clearly shown to be untrue. Although snorting cocaine may be less addicting than smoking freebase or "crack" or injecting cocaine intravenously, this does not in any way make it safe. For example, 49 percent of the cocaine addicts admitted to our hospital unit have been exclusively intranasal users. A study of 136 cocaine abusers admitted to a Colorado drug abuse facility showed similar statistics: 57 percent of their patients were intranasal users. Thus, "merely" snorting cocaine offers no protection against the serious consequences of the drug.

Smoking Cocaine

A second method by which cocaine can be used is by smoking. Cocaine can be smoked either as coca paste, which is currently gaining great popularity in South America, or as cocaine freebase, which is much more popular in the United States. A recently introduced form of cocaine, known as "crack," is cocaine freebase sold in ready-to-smoke form.

Coca Paste

The practice of smoking coca paste first received attention in the early 1970s when Peruvian doctors began to see an increasing number of young people who were experiencing severe physical and psychological difficulties as a result of repetitive smoking. Many of these individuals were hospitalized because of compulsive use of the drug, while others died as the result of acute cocaine intoxication.

Coca paste consists of a mixture of cocaine, kerosene, sulfuric acid, and sodium carbonate. The purity of the paste may vary widely; laboratory analyses have revealed concentrations of cocaine ranging from 40 to 91 percent. The white or brown paste is allowed to dry after being manufactured from the aforementioned ingredients; it is then placed at the end of a tobacco or marijuana cigarette, ignited, and inhaled deeply.

Coca paste is absorbed into the blood very rapidly after smoking; studies of healthy volunteers have shown that the blood level of cocaine after smoking paste rises as rapidly as after intravenous injection of the drug. Physical effects include increased pulse, blood pressure, respiratory rate, and body temperature. Dilated pupils, muscle tension, tremulousness, and heavy perspiration are also common effects of the drug. Although initial use of the drug is characterized by euphoria, gregariousness, and a sense of well-being, repeated exposure frequently causes anxiety, hostility, and extreme depression. As people smoke more heavily, the period of euphoria may last for only a few seconds, followed by anxiety and a craving for more cocaine. Long-term users may also drink alcohol in order to decrease their anxiety and alter the rapidly changing moods caused by coca paste.

Further use of coca paste can lead to a wide variety of symptoms: numbness in the mouth, a burning sensation in the eyes, pounding heartbeat, tremulous limbs, headache, insomnia, dizziness, abdominal pain, and profuse sweating. Continued use may lead to visual and auditory misperceptions, as harmless objects and noises may begin to appear threatening. Feelings of anxiety may become overwhelming, and these are sometimes accompanied by aggressiveness or severe depression. Hallucinations may occur if the drug use continues; the long-term smoker may hear, see, feel, or smell things that are not there, and he may become frankly paranoid. Individuals continuing to smoke the drug may develop "coca paste psychosis," characterized by extreme hypervigilance, paranoid delusions, and hallucinations. This is an extremely serious condition in which overdoses, suicides, and homicides have occurred.

Unfortunately, the attempts to treat compulsive coca paste smoking in South America have often been unsuccessful; relapse rates are high and the consequences of ongoing coca paste smoking can be grave.

Smoking Cocaine Freebase or Crack

The most common form of cocaine smoking in the United States is "freebasing": smoking alkaloidal cocaine, or freebase. Freebasing first attracted the attention of American cocaine users in the mid-1970s and has continued to gain popularity since.

Freebase is prepared by dissolving cocaine hydrochloride in water and then adding a strong base such as ammonia or baking soda to this aqueous solution. This chemical process produces cocaine freebase, which may be dissolved in ether to extract the cocaine. The ether is then removed by drying, resulting in a product which may range from 37 to 96 percent purity. An alternate method of preparation bypasses the ether; in this process, the mixture of cocaine and alkali is washed and filtered instead of adding ether.

A recently developed form of freebase, known as "crack" (or "rock"), is cocaine freebase that has been manufactured from cocaine hydrochloride by the dealer rather than by the user. The resultant product consists of small chips that resemble white pebbles; these "rocks" of ready-to-smoke freebase may be sold for as little as $10 each, and may contain in excess of 75 percent pure cocaine. The low price, ease of use, high purity, and extremely addictive nature of crack portend a frightening scenario of increasing cocaine use and addiction in the near future, particularly among adolescents.

One difference between cocaine freebase (or crack) and coca paste is the fact that the former preparation does not contain some of the solvents, such as kerosene, which are present in the paste. The method of administration is also different. Although freebase can, like paste, be added to a tobacco or marijuana cigarette, it is usually placed on a series of screens in the neck of a water pipe. The drug is then ignited and deeply inhaled, as in marijuana and coca paste smoking. Although the drug paraphernalia industry has devised increasingly sophisticated equipment in order to capture higher yields of pure drug from freebasing, inhalation from a water pipe is typically accompanied by the loss of a great deal of cocaine. In fact, some studies have shown that only 1 to 5 percent of the initial cocaine is actually inhaled by this method. Smoking freebase cocaine through a cigarette is similarly inefficient; nearly half of the cocaine is lost through the burning end of the cigarette, and only about 6 percent is inhaled. The inefficiency of freebase smoking is one of the factors that makes this form of cocaine abuse so expensive.

Freebase or crack smoking causes a very rapid rise in the blood level of cocaine and produces almost instantaneous psychological effects, which peak in about five minutes. After a typical dose ("hit") of 50 to 150 milligrams, the user will experience intense euphoria almost immediately, accompanied by a rise in blood pressure, pulse, body temperature, and respiratory rate. A research study conducted by Dr. M. Perez-Reyes at the University of North Carolina revealed that the psychological and physical effects of freebase smoking were as powerful as those produced by an injection of intravenous cocaine. The euphoria produced by smoking is quite short-lived, however, ending 10 to 20 minutes after inhalation. Although some freebase or crack smokers experience little in the way of after-effects, many become quite anxious and depressed after the drug has worn off; these feelings are sometimes accompanied by severe drug craving. Indeed, Dr. Perez-Reyes found that freebase smokers reported a higher degree of craving for cocaine following drug use than did intravenous users.

Some of the characteristics of freebase or crack that make it so addictive include the intensity of euphoria it produces, its nearly immediate onset of action, and the rapidity with which its effects disappear. In addition, the aftermath of freebasing is often characterized by severe craving for more drug. Although some individuals may stop after limiting themselves to one or two "hits," repetitive use is a much more common pattern. Since the psychological effects of freebasing peak five minutes after use, only to be followed by severe depression, agitation, and drug craving ("crashing") 10 minutes later, many free-basers try to ward off these symptoms by smoking again before they occur. Since the period of time between intoxication and crashing is so short, these individuals may end up smoking cocaine almost continuously, remaining in a nearly constant state of intoxication until the drug supply has been exhausted. This pattern of cocaine use is called a "run," and may last from several hours to a number of days. The addictive nature of freebasing, coupled with its inefficiency, can lead to a very expensive habit. We have treated some freebase smokers who have described runs lasting up to two weeks, during which they smoked up to an ounce of cocaine (street price: approximately $2000) each day.

Many of the symptoms produced by long-term freebase or crack smoking are similar to those described above for the coca paste smokers. In addition, other hazards have been reported. For example, the combination of extremely intoxicated users, open flames, and volatile chemicals such as ether creates the potential for disastrous explosions or fires. In addition, long-term cocaine smoking may cause lung malfunction. In 1981, we collaborated with researchers from the Department of Pulmonary (Lung) Medicine at Massachusetts General Hospital in Boston, reporting lung dysfunction in two freebase smokers. Since that time, we have continued to study the effects of freebase smoking on the lungs, and we have found impaired lung function in many of these individuals when compared with a normal population. Moreover, a group of researchers at Northwestern University recently published a report in which over half of the freebase smokers they tested had similar difficulties. Thus, there appears to be mounting evidence that freebase smoking may be harmful to the lungs.

Intravenous Cocaine Use

Perhaps the most perilous method of cocaine administration is intravenous use of the drug. In addition to its high addiction liability (much like freebase or crack smoking), intravenous use carries with it the additional hazard of unsterile needles. Intravenous use is a more common method of cocaine administration in addicts than in occasional users. Since taking poor care of oneself is frequently part of the addictive process, many severe cocaine abusers share needles and expose themselves to serious medical complications, in particular hepatitis, endocarditis, and acquired immune deficiency syndrome (AIDS). These diseases are discussed in Chapter 3.

Cocaine is prepared for intravenous administration by placing between one-tenth and one-quarter of a gram in a spoon, and then adding water. This aqueous solution is then strained, after which it is drawn up into a syringe and injected into a vein. Euphoria occurs almost immediately.

With more frequent use, some individuals gradually increase their dosage of cocaine, so that they may inject up to a gram at a time. Like freebase or crack smokers, intravenous users frequently take cocaine in sprees ("runs"): discrete episodes of highly intensive drug use. During these periods, they may use massive amounts of cocaine, perhaps spending thousands of dollars in a week. A study by Drs. Frank Gawin and Herbert Kleber at the Yale University School of Medicine showed that while intravenous and intranasal cocaine abusers both took similar amounts of cocaine when averaged out over a week, the former group tended to use very large amounts of cocaine in discrete, brief periods, while the intranasal users took the drug more often but in lower doses. Freebase smokers in their study used almost twice as much cocaine as the other two groups, with longer runs and even heavier drug use than the intravenous users.

Intravenous use of cocaine is highly addictive for the same reasons that we discussed for freebase or crack smoking: the intensity of the euphoria, the nearly immediate onset of action, and the brevity of the "high." An intravenous user may become depressed and irritable within five to 15 minutes after drug use.

This "crash" frequently leads to frantic repeated injections, sometimes occurring as often as every five minutes. This scenario was described by one patient:

> Once I started shooting coke, my life became a complete nightmare. It was as if I was a slave to the needle. Within literally a couple of minutes after sticking the needle into my arm, I was a basket case. I would stand around sweating and shaking, and I'd be paranoid that the police were going to break into my house. The worst part was that in spite of all this, I couldn't wait to "boot" [inject] more coke. That needle became my entire world. By the end of a run, I'd be stabbing myself all over the place looking for a vein, getting sloppier each time. There would be blood dripping all over the floor, all over my clothes, all over everything, and I didn't care at all.

A relatively recent phenomenon among intravenous cocaine users is "speedballing," which involves mixing cocaine and heroin and injecting them together. The purpose of this practice is to buffer ("mellow out") the stimulant effects of cocaine with the more sedating, relaxing effects of heroin. In addition, the longer-lasting opiate effect helps to guard against the depression that frequently follows cocaine use. Some users believe that the combination of an "upper" (cocaine) and a "downer" (heroin) makes the combination safer than either of the two drugs taken individually. Unfortunately, this presumption is untrue; the potentially fatal respiratory depression caused by heroin may be made more severe by cocaine, thus rendering the combination of cocaine and heroin even more dangerous than the use of either drug alone.

As we will discuss in Chapter 3, one of the major hazards of intravenous cocaine use is the risk involved in using unsterile needles. Insulin syringes (legally sold by prescription only) are typically sold on the street for approximately $3 each, although the price can go much higher in some areas. However, as for any other commodity, the price is dictated in part by the quality of the product. Thus, used needles are sold more cheaply than new, sterile needles. The most desperate addicts and those with the fewest financial resources are thus most likely to use contaminated needles. They therefore carry a higher risk of acquiring and spreading needle-related infections.

3

The Effects of Cocaine
on the Body

In discussing the effects of cocaine on the body, it is important to keep in mind that street preparations of cocaine have been adulterated with a variety of "cuts" (see Table 1), all of which are designed to dilute the amount of pure cocaine being sold and thus increase the profit to the seller. Since the product advertised as "cocaine" may contain as little as 10 percent pure drug, the potential physical problems resulting from street cocaine will depend in part on the specific cuts being used and will therefore exceed the list of complications presented here.

When cocaine is taken into the body either intranasally, intravenously, by smoking, or through other mucous membranes including the vagina, gums, or urethra, the drug is taken up by a large number of body organs, including the liver, kidney, heart, and brain. Much of the drug also penetrates into fat tissue. The blood level of cocaine is highest approximately five minutes after smoking or taking the drug intravenously; peak blood levels tend to occur 15 to 60 minutes after snorting.

Cocaine is broken down quickly by the body into inactive by-products and is largely eliminated within 24 hours. The drug appears to be broken down largely by an enzyme in the blood called pseudocholinesterase. This information is important because there is a small number of people who are born with a deficiency of this enzyme. This problem would not otherwise

Table 1. Common Adulterants ("Cuts") Used to Dilute Cocaine

Sugars	Miscellaneous Fillers
Lactose	Cornstarch
Glucose	Flour
Mannitol	Talc
Inositol	Phencyclidine (PCP)
	Heroin
Other Local Anesthetics	Quinine
Lidocaine	
Tetracaine	
Procaine	
Benzocaine	

be detected except through the administration of certain general anesthetics that are also broken down by the same enzyme. Thus, an individual with a pseudocholinesterase deficiency might have a severe toxic or even fatal reaction to even a small amount of cocaine, since the ordinarily rapid breakdown of the drug cannot occur. Cocaine is metabolized into a number of by-products, some of them active and others inactive. The compound most commonly detected in people's urine is called benzoylecgonine; this metabolite can be detected for up to several days after cocaine use.

The General Physical Effects of Cocaine

The major medical use for cocaine today is as a local anesthetic in ear, nose, and throat surgery. Cocaine was, in fact, the first local anesthetic, having initially been used in eye surgery a century ago. The reason cocaine is still preferred as a local anesthetic in some surgical procedures is its ability to constrict blood vessels in the area to which it has been applied. This "vasoconstrictor" effect decreases bleeding during surgery, thus allowing the surgeon to see the operative field more clearly. Since the ear, nose, and throat contain many blood vessels, cocaine is a particularly valuable anesthetic in this type of surgery. We will discuss later how cocaine-induced vasoconstriction can cause problems when the drug is repeatedly applied to the nose or, in the case of freebasing, the lungs.

Another major effect of cocaine is its activation of the sympathetic nervous system, which controls numerous functions of the brain and other organs, including blood pressure, heart rate, contractility of heart muscle, blood sugar level, mood, and appetite. The sympathetic nervous system is the part of the body which, among other functions, controls the "fight or flight" response. When a person experiences danger or other significant stress, the sympathetic nervous system can respond by triggering the release of certain hormones (predominantly epinephrine) and neurotransmitters (such as norepinephrine and dopamine) that help the body respond to the danger. When the sympathetic nervous system is activated, the heart pumps faster and more powerfully in order to increase the flow of blood in critical areas. Blood pressure rises, body temperature increases, and the individual becomes more activated and alert. The need for food and sleep diminishes, since—in an evolutionary sense—these activities only interfere with the need to fight or run. By activating the sympathetic nervous system, cocaine causes euphoria, decreased appetite, mental stimulation, rapid heartbeat, increased blood pressure, elevated body temperature, an increased rate of breathing, more rapid brain electrical activity, and an elevated blood sugar level. Although some of these effects are generally sought out by cocaine users, an excess of these physiological responses can precipitate significant problems.

Medical Complications from Cocaine

The adverse medical effects that may result from using street cocaine can be divided into several major categories (see Table 2).

First, complications may occur immediately as the result of taking too much cocaine—that is, an overdose. Second, there are long-term effects that occur as the result of repeated cocaine use. In addition to the direct results of the drug, medical complications in cocaine users may be caused by paraphernalia (in particular, unsterile needles) or adulterants ("cuts"). Finally, long-term cocaine abusers frequently develop psychiatric problems and engage in a life-style that may increase their risk to develop certain medical complications.

Table 2. Medical Complications from Cocaine

I. Drug Effects
  A. Overdose
   1. Rapid irregular heartbeat (ventricular tachycardia or fibrillation)
   2. Cerebral hemorrhage
   3. Seizures
   4. Heat stroke
   5. Respiratory failure
  B. Chronic Nasal Problems
   1. Chronic nasal congestion and cold symptoms
   2. Frequent nosebleeds
   3. Ulcerations of nose
   4. Perforation of nasal septum
  C. Lung Damage from Freebase Smoking
  D. Vitamin B and C Deficiencies

II. Complications Due to Paraphernalia
  A. Unsterile Needles
   1. Skin infections
   2. Hepatitis
   3. Endocarditis
   4. Acquired immune deficiency syndrome (AIDS)
  B. Freebase Paraphernalia (torches and volatile chemicals)
   1. Explosions, burns

III. Complications Due to Adulterants ("Cuts")
  A. Inflammation in lungs
  B. Virtually anything, depending upon the adulterant

IV. Complications Due to Psychiatric Effects and Life-Style
  A. Suicide
  B. Accidents
  C. Homicide

Cocaine Overdose

Fifteen years ago, deaths from cocaine overdose were rarely seen. It was widely assumed that the only people who died from cocaine use were drug traffickers and large-scale dealers who were known to smuggle large amounts of cocaine by placing it in condoms and swallowing them before boarding an airplane. If the condoms ruptured, massive quantities of cocaine would be released into the bloodstreams of these individuals, frequently killing them while still airborne.

Death from cocaine overdose is no longer confined to drug smugglers, however. Rather, an excess of cocaine was involved in one-sixth of all drug-related cases seen by medical examiners in 1984. Although intravenous use carries the highest risk of fatal overdose, freebase or crack smokers and intranasal users are also in jeopardy.

How Cocaine Can Kill

The lethal effects of cocaine represent an exaggeration of the typical physical effects produced by the drug. Thus, there are many mechanisms by which cocaine can cause a fatal overdose.

1. Cocaine increases heart rate. If one's heart beats too rapidly, the steady rhythm of the heart may be disturbed, and irregular electrical activity may occur. Indeed, feeling one's heart "skipping a beat" is one of the most common reactions that cocaine users experience. Abnormal heart rhythm may be quite dangerous in certain individuals and may quickly lead to a dangerous heart irregularity known as ventricular tachycardia (extremely rapid, although regular contraction of the heart) or ventricular fibrillation (irregular and very weak motions of the heart): either of these conditions can be quickly fatal.
2. The ability of cocaine to increase blood pressure can also cause trouble; if one's blood pressure increases too rapidly or too much, a weak-walled blood vessel in the brain may burst under increased pressure, causing a cerebral hemorrhage (bleeding into the brain). This type of stroke is often fatal.

3. The increased body temperature that cocaine causes may occasionally reach dangerous heights in certain individuals; this complication is known as hyperpyrexia.

4. Cocaine use can precipitate grand mal seizures (epileptic convulsions), sometimes at relatively low doses. Indeed, long-term cocaine use may eventually sensitize the individual to further seizures at increasingly lower doses, a phenomenon known medically as "kindling." Although grand mal seizures are not in themselves always life-threatening, they may be fatal under some circumstances. For example, several seizures may occur rapidly in succession, a very serious and sometimes fatal condition known as status epilepticus. A seizure may also occur at an inopportune moment, such as while driving a car or crossing the street. Clearly, fatalities can also occur at these times.

5. Respiratory difficulties are another cause of cocaine-related deaths. As a user increases his dose of cocaine, the deep rapid respirations that often occur after low to moderate doses may give way to labored breathing; an overdose may produce gasping, shallow irregular breaths that can culminate in respiratory arrest (cessation of breathing).

6. Cocaine overdoses may also occur in special populations. We have already mentioned the rare individuals who are born with a deficiency of pseudocholinesterase, an enzyme that breaks down cocaine. Deaths have been reported in such individuals who have been given as little as 20 milligrams of cocaine as a local anesthetic. Cocaine may also increase levels of blood sugar, thus harming patients with diabetes. Individuals with angina pectoris (chest pain due to coronary artery disease) may also aggravate their condition through cocaine use. Indeed, some such patients have experienced a fatal reaction to cocaine because their heart muscles were forced to work beyond the ability of their diseased coronary arteries to supply them with oxygen.

Some people want to know a "safe" way to use cocaine. Unfortunately, there is no clear answer to this. Individuals vary in their sensitivity to the drug, so a dose that may be "safe" in one person may precipitate severe medical difficulties or even death in another. For example, individuals with pseudocho-linesterase deficiency can have severe reactions to even minute doses of cocaine. It is thus reasonable to conclude that there is no predictably safe dose of cocaine.

Effects of Long-Term Cocaine Use

The medical complications that may occur as the result of repeated cocaine use can be divided into several major categories. First is the group of complications that occur because of the repeated use of cocaine itself. The other medical problems develop as the result of the adulterants ("cuts"), drug paraphernalia (e.g., unsterile needles), psychiatric symptoms or life-style that generally accompany cocaine use.

Medical Complications Due to Effects of Cocaine Itself

Nose Problems

The area most often damaged by intranasal cocaine use is the site where cocaine enters the body—the nose. As we mentioned before, cocaine is a very powerful vasoconstrictor. Thus, blood vessels in the area exposed to cocaine are reduced in size, and blood flow to that area is diminished. Since the blood transports oxygen and other nutrients required to keep body tissues alive and healthy, an area that is repeatedly exposed to cocaine will, in essence, be malnourished. Thus, the mucous membranes of the nose may become irritated and inflamed, and painful ulcers may develop inside the nostrils. Chronic sneezing, frequent nosebleeds, and nasal congestion are common symptoms. Experienced cocaine users frequently try to avert these consequences by rinsing their nasal passages with salt water or by applying glycerin, vitamin E, or petroleum jelly (Vaseline) to their noses. However, these home remedies are generally unsuccessful, and they are frequently applied less often as cocaine use increases.

Long-term intranasal cocaine use can sometimes lead to tissue death and eventual perforation of the nasal septum (the portion of the nose that separates the two nostrils). Although

still relatively uncommon, perforated nasal septa are now being seen more frequently in drug abuse treatment centers; the
only treatment available is plastic surgery.

Lung Problems

In addition to the immediate danger of respiratory arrest
from a fatal overdose of cocaine, recent evidence has begun to
reveal some of the long-term medical hazards associated with
long-term cocaine smoking. Indeed, in collaboration with pulmonary (lung) physicians at Massachusetts General Hospital,
we have discovered that the lungs of freebase smokers frequently show a decreased ability to perform one of their major
tasks: the transportation of oxygen into the blood. We have
explained our findings by hypothesizing that the vasoconstrictor effect of cocaine, which causes so much obvious damage in
the nostrils of intranasal users, may impair pulmonary function by causing similar changes in the blood vessels of the
lungs.

Recently, a group of researchers at Northwestern University
Medical School have reported similar respiratory abnormalities in 10 of the 19 patients they studied. Thus, evidence is
gradually mounting to indicate that freebase smoking may lead
to serious lung dysfunction. Moreover, in some individuals,
this process may occur after a relatively short smoking history;
impairment of lung function has been reported in individuals
who have smoked freebase for as little as three months.

Vitamin Deficiencies

One of the prominent effects of cocaine is its ability to sup-
press appetite and cause weight loss. For many users, this property is highly desirable. Frequently accompanying the weight
loss, however, is a deficiency of vitamins, particularly the wa-
ter-soluble B and C vitamins. Indeed, Dr. Mark Gold reported
that 19 of 26 cocaine abusers hospitalized at Fair Oaks Hospital
in Summit, New Jersey, were deficient in at least one vitamin,
with vitamin B6 (pyridoxine) deficiency being most common.
In addition to causing vitamin deficiencies, the weight loss that
often accompanies long-term cocaine use may result in other

manifestations of malnutrition, including anemia and metabolic abnormalities.

Seizures (Convulsions)

One of the most dangerous complications of cocaine use is grand mal seizures, such as those that occur in people who have epilepsy. Seizures occur as a result of the uncontrolled release of electrical discharges in the brain. Since cocaine reduces the threshold for seizures, vulnerable individuals may suffer a convulsion after just a single dose of cocaine. For others, repeated use of cocaine may gradually lower the seizure threshold. This "kindling" effect may eventually lead to the development of seizures, which can be extremely dangerous and are sometimes fatal.

Sexual Difficulties

One frequently cited reason for cocaine use is its reputation as an aphrodisiac. This perception was not confirmed, however, in a study of regular cocaine users by UCLA psychologist Ronald Siegel; he found that only 13 percent of those surveyed claimed to experience increased sexual stimulation from cocaine use. Although the mental stimulation and disinhibition from cocaine may initially heighten sexual pleasure, higher doses and more frequent drug use generally lead to sexual dysfunction. Impotence and inability to ejaculate are common complaints in male cocaine users; decreased desire for sex becomes the norm in users of both sexes. Some people who initially find sex more pleasurable while intoxicated may become dependent on the use of cocaine for sexual arousal; they may even find themselves unable to enjoy sex at all for a long period of time following long-term cocaine use.

Some cocaine users attempt to increase their sexual pleasure by directly applying the drug to their genitals. Since cocaine is a local anesthetic, placement of the drug on a mucous membrane such as the penis or clitoris may in fact decrease sensation and prolong sexual intercourse. Unfortunately, this practice can be quite hazardous, since the tissues to which cocaine has been applied may receive decreased blood flow and may dry up and become ulcerated.

Adverse Effects on Pregnancy

Physicians have long suspected that cocaine may harm the fetus; a 1985 study by Dr. Ira Chasnoff and his colleagues at Northwestern University Medical School confirmed this suspicion. These researchers found an abnormally high rate of spontaneous abortion (miscarriage) and abruptio placentae (premature separation of the placenta) in women who used cocaine during pregnancy. In addition, many of the infants born to these women were more tremulous and less interactive than normal babies.

Medical Complications Due to Drug Paraphernalia

Many of the medical difficulties that cocaine users experience are not caused by cocaine itself. Rather, they occur as a result of other factors that are as much a part of illicit cocaine use as the drug itself: drug paraphernalia and adulterants. The most hazardous of all drug paraphernalia is the unsterile needle. A needle is sterile if it is used only once after direct removal from a sterile package. Although this is the only method used in clinical medicine, sterile technique is uncommon in illicit drug users. Rather, the rule among cocaine abusers and other intravenous drug users is to use the same needle and syringe (commonly referred to as "a set of works") repeatedly, because they are often expensive and sometimes difficult to obtain. An even more dangerous, but very common, method of needle use is that of sharing needles with other drug users. This practice can lead to a variety of very serious illnesses, including hepatitis and acquired immune deficiency syndrome (AIDS).

Skin Infections

Perhaps the most common medical problem seen in intravenous cocaine abusers is infection of the skin and the tissues underneath the skin near injection sites. This occurs because an unsterile needle introduces bacteria underneath the outer layer of the skin, which normally acts as the body's first line of defense against infection. The introduction of bacteria into deeper layers of the skin may serve as a focus for infection. The most common manifestations of a skin infection include redness, swelling, heat, pain, and tenderness in the infected area. Spread of the infection may be detected by red streaks under the skin, signifying that the infection has spread to the lymphatic channels. If the infection is accompanied by fever, rapid heartbeat, and chills, then it may have spread into the bloodstream. This is an extremely serious sign, requiring immediate treatment, for it is potentially fatal if untreated.

Although skin infections may seem rather benign, they deserve prompt medical attention because of their ability to spread rather quickly and cause serious damage both locally (e.g., infection of the tendon, joint, or bone) and in the rest of the body. Treatment for skin infections may consist of rest, moist heat, antibiotics, surgical drainage, or a combination of these treatments.

Hepatitis

Hepatitis, or inflammation of the liver, is another very common disorder in cocaine abusers, particularly intravenous users. A New York study estimated that approximately two-thirds of intravenous drug abusers develop hepatitis at some point in their drug abusing careers; two-thirds of this subpopulation contracts the disease within the first two years after injecting drugs. Thus, the chance of an intravenous cocaine abuser developing hepatitis is approximately 50 percent within the first two years of drug use. Whereas hepatitis can be caused by a variety of agents—including alcohol, certain general anesthetics, and toxic chemicals—the most common form in cocaine abusers is caused by a virus that is transmitted from the blood of one user to that of another. Thus, hepatitis in cocaine abusers usually occurs as a result of sharing paraphernalia with other individuals who are already infected. Although the most common vehicle for the transmission of hepatitis in this population is a needle, there have been reports of hepatitis in exclusively intranasal cocaine abusers, perhaps caused by sharing straws, dollar bills, or "tooters" (thin glass or metal cylinders used for snorting cocaine) with other users. Since nosebleeds are commonly seen in active cocaine users, blood can easily be transmitted from one cocaine snorter to another;

it takes less than a drop of contaminated blood to infect another person with hepatitis.

The most serious form of hepatitis in drug users is hepatitis
B, formerly termed "serum hepatitis." One reason for the
name change is the fact that hepatitis B can be transmitted via
other means besides blood, such as through intimate sexual
contact. However, infections in intravenous cocaine abusers
are probably blood-borne in most cases. The disease is transmitted as follows: John, already infected with the hepatitis B
virus, injects cocaine. Upon inserting the needle into his vein,
the virus in his bloodstream contaminates the needle. This
needle is then shared with Susan, who then injects the virus
into her bloodstream along with her cocaine. After an incubation period ranging from one to six months (average is two to
three months), the disease may strike.

Early symptoms of hepatitis vary widely and may include
nausea, vomiting, headache, sore throat, cough, decreased appetite, fatigue, or joint pains. Patients with hepatitis often complain of an altered sense of taste or smell; cigarette smokers
may find that smoking becomes unenjoyable because of the
change in their taste sensation. Patients may experience a dark-
ening of their urine and/or a lightening of their stools, which
may appear clay colored. An enlargement of the liver may
occur during hepatitis; the liver, which is located under the
right side of the rib cage, may become quite tender, especially
during deep breathing. Jaundice, a yellow coloration of the
skin or the whites of the eyes, may occur. Although this is
considered by many drug users to be the hallmark of hepatitis,
a significant number of patients with hepatitis never become
jaundiced. Indeed, some people infected with the virus remain
totally asymptomatic. Many intravenous users attempt to "protect" themselves against hepatitis by refusing to share a needle
with a jaundiced drug user. Unfortunately, however, this rule of
thumb is not an effective means of preventing hepatitis, both
because of the long incubation period of hepatitis B (during
which time the patient may be asymptomatic but highly infectious), and because jaundice is not uniformly seen in patients
with hepatitis.

Recovery from hepatitis B generally occurs within two to 12
weeks, although fatigue may occur for even longer. Although

the death rate from hepatitis B is estimated at less than 1 percent, chronic hepatitis may develop in up to 10 percent of all cases. Chronic hepatitis may progress to cirrhosis, a scarring of the liver that is sometimes fatal.

Hepatitis B is not the only form of liver disease that occurs in cocaine users. Another form of hepatitis, referred to as non-A, non-B hepatitis, is also commonly seen among intravenous drug users. The disease is designated "non-A, non-B" because there are many cases of hepatitis that appear to be viral in origin, but for which no virus can be found on blood examination. Hepatitis A, which is transmitted through fecal material, is not necessarily more common in drug abusers than in other individuals. Non-A, non-B hepatitis, however, appears to be transmitted like hepatitis B.

Once an individual has developed hepatitis B, he generally develops antibodies to fight off the virus. This antibody may then provide protection against reinfection with the hepatitis B virus. Unfortunately, protection against hepatitis B does not provide immunity against future infection with non-A, non-B hepatitis. Many intravenous drug users are under the mistaken impression that after having hepatitis, they are henceforth immune to the disease. This is not true. Continued use of unsterile needles may result in repeated episodes of non-A, non-B hepatitis.

About 1 percent of individuals with hepatitis B do not develop antibodies and remain chronic carriers of the virus— that is, they remain chronically infectious. This chronic carrier state may or may not be associated with chronic hepatitis.

Treatment and Prevention of Viral Hepatitis. There is no specific treatment for acute viral hepatitis. For individuals who have recently been exposed to the hepatitis B virus, an injection of hepatitis B immune globulin (HBIG) may be recommended in order to decrease the likelihood and seriousness of the disease. Otherwise, the best advice is to eat and sleep well and to avoid contact with alcohol (a liver toxin) and needles. In 1982, a hepatitis B vaccine was developed. The vaccine, which consists of highly purified, inactivated hepatitis B antigen obtained from the blood of chronic carriers, appears to offer excellent protection against hepatitis B, although it is unclear whether long-term side effects will appear as we gain more experience with the vaccine. It is also not clear how long the vaccine will provide protection.

Acquired Immune Deficiency Syndrome (AIDS)

In 1981, the medical community first filed reports of a heretofore unreported syndrome. Previously healthy homosexual men were developing an extremely rare tumor known as Kaposi's sarcoma, and a form of pneumonia (*Pneumocystis carinii*) that is generally seen only in patients with severely compromised immune systems. Since that time, thousands of similar cases have been reported concerning individuals whose immune systems have been overwhelmed. To date, this disease, known as acquired immune deficiency syndrome (AIDS), has been almost uniformly fatal. Nearly one-fifth of those afflicted with AIDS are intravenous drug abusers. Next to male homosexuals, intravenous drug abusers are the group at highest risk of contracting AIDS. AIDS appears to be a viral infection, caused by the human T-cell lymphotropic virus (HTLV-III). Most researchers posit that AIDS, like hepatitis B, is transmitted via blood or intimate sexual contact. The incubation period in AIDS is thought to be quite long, possibly several years or longer. Although a blood test is currently available to determine whether an individual has antibodies to HTLV-III, it is unclear how many people with a positive test will actually develop the disease. Thus far, there is no known treatment for the underlying immune defect in AIDS. As of this time, the three-year survival rate for the disease is less than 10 percent.

Endocarditis

Endocarditis, an infection of the heart valve, is one of the most serious infections that can develop in intravenous cocaine abusers. The disease develops when bacteria enter the bloodstream via unsterile needles and are deposited on a heart valve, where they may begin to multiply. These bacteria may then travel from the heart to other areas of the body, where they can cause great harm. For example, a shower of bacteria that lands in the lungs may cause a septic clot in the lung (pulmonary embolus), while a similar event in the brain may cause a stroke and a brain abscess.

When endocarditis occurs in an intravenous drug user, the disease usually occurs acutely and progresses rapidly. High fever and chills are common. Abscesses may occur in the lungs, brain, or kidneys. When untreated, endocarditis is usually fatal. Some intravenous drug users, particularly heroin addicts, may misinterpret the fever and chills of endocarditis, believing that they are experiencing drug withdrawal. Many intravenous drug users ignore such manifestations of physical illness because of a general pattern of self-neglect and because of suspiciousness of physicians and hospitals. However, with appropriate treatment, which usually consists of at least four weeks of intravenous antibiotics, recovery may occur. The involved valve or valves may nevertheless sustain damage, perhaps necessitating surgical valve replacement at some future date.

Burns

One of the most dangerous aspects of cocaine freebase smoking is the risk of fire or explosion. One preparation process for freebase makes occasional disastrous accidents inevitable, as highly intoxicated individuals make use of open flames in combination with highly flammable volatile solvents such as ether.

Medical Complications Due to Adulterants ("Cuts")

Lung Damage

Although cocaine itself can produce a wide variety of medical and psychological problems in its users, street "cocaine" presents additional hazards. Since illicitly purchased cocaine may be as little as 10 percent pure, up to 90 percent of the product being snorted, smoked, or injected is present only because it either looks, tastes, or feels like cocaine. These adulterants (cuts) can cause much of the toxicity that cocaine users experience.

One of the problems that intravenous drug users frequently encounter is lung damage due to the frequent injection of adulterants such as talc or starch. Researchers have hypothesized that the injection of these adulterants obstructs small blood vessels in the lungs, causing an inflammatory reaction in the lungs (granulomatous lung disease). This is typically a persistent, smoldering area of inflammation that may last for months or longer, even after the cessation of drug use. It has been estimated that 25 to 70 percent of intravenous drug abusers have such abnormalities in their lungs. These abnormalities can occur even in the absence of symptoms (e.g., shortness of breath or cough) that one would ordinarily expect in patients with lung disease.

Medical Complications Due to Life-Style and Psychiatric Symptoms in Cocaine Abusers

Suicide

Another group of health hazards resulting from long-term cocaine use occurs because of the psychiatric effects of cocaine and the life-style that frequently accompanies its use. As we have discussed, cocaine can cause roller-coaster-like swings between euphoria and depression. As the frequency and intensity of cocaine use increase, the severity of the depression can increase proportionately. Some cocaine abusers become suicidal as a result of the neurochemical depression caused by the drug and because of the sense of hopelessness that they may experience after repeated unsuccessful attempts to stop their drug use. Thus, the risk of suicide represents another potential medical danger in cocaine abusers.

Accidents

In addition to the accidental deaths that can occur as the result of an unintentional overdose, automobile accidents are much more likely to occur among long-term cocaine abusers. Although data supporting this are not as readily available as statistics concerning driving while under the influence of alcohol, the sense of invincibility that cocaine users often feel may encourage them to drive faster and more recklessly than they ordinarily would. This can occur even in occasional users and is not merely the result of long-term cocaine abuse. Drunk driving may be a secondary consequence of cocaine use, as many individuals attempt to "smooth out" their "high" by using other drugs such as alcohol, Valium, barbiturates, Quaalude, marijuana, or heroin, all of which have been very clearly shown to impair driving ability.

Homicide

A final cause of death in cocaine abusers is murder. Homicide may occur for several reasons. First, cocaine is illegal. Thus, in order to obtain cocaine, one must deal with criminals. Although some cocaine abusers initially buy their drugs from friends in small quantities, the dangerousness of their contacts often increases as their drug habit escalates. Many prospective cocaine buyers frequently enter into dangerous situations while carrying large sums of money, thus presenting inviting targets for robbery, mugging, or murder. In addition, since large doses of cocaine often produce paranoia, heavy users may attempt to defend themselves against real or imagined enemies by obtaining weapons. Such was the case with John, a 27-year-old man who had been using cocaine for two years.

> After a while, I was convinced that there were people trying to break into my house. I didn't know who they were, but I was sure that people were after me. There was probably some reality to it too, since I really was scared that the police would come in and bust me. The only way that I felt that I could protect myself was by getting a knife. So I started sleeping with a butcher knife next to me. That didn't work for long, though, because I still felt insecure. So I felt that I had to get a gun. Every night, I went to bed with a gun on one side of me and a butcher knife on the other side. I was just waiting for someone to come in the house so that I could blow his brains out. God knows what I was going to do with the knife. I swear, I was a maniac. It wouldn't have mattered who had come to the door. If someone had come to my door at the wrong time to borrow a cup of sugar, I can tell you with 100 percent certainty, he would have been dead.

Clearly, a man such as John, whose story is not unusual, is also a target for other paranoid cocaine abusers with whom he

is dealing. This combination of extremely poor judgment, paranoia, intermittent crippling depression, and a stockpiling of
lethal weapons may lead to violent deaths in an unfortunate
number of long-term cocaine abusers.

4

Cocaine and the Brain

The widespread popularity of cocaine reflects the drug's powerful effects on the brain and, consequently, on behavior. However, although cocaine is highly valued for its ability to produce euphoria, enhance alertness, and alleviate fatigue, most users think very little about the drug's long-term effects on mood. In this chapter we will describe both the short- and long-term effects of cocaine on brain function. This information is based on research carried out on both animal and human subjects, as well as on the accumulated experience of over 1500 years of cocaine consumption.

Basic Elements of Brain Function: The Nerve Cell

Understanding the effects of cocaine (or any drug) on brain function first requires some knowledge about how the brain works. The brain consists of a collection of nerve cells called *neurons*, which are unique among all cells of the body in that they are specially adapted to receive and dispatch electrical impulses. Neurons are able to accomplish this because of their unique anatomical and physiological characteristics.

As shown in Figure 1, the typical nerve cell has a system of branches, called *dendrites*, whose specialized surfaces are equipped to receive incoming electrical signals from other

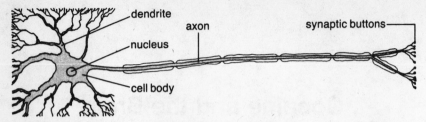

Figure 1. Diagram of a typical nerve cell. (Illustration by David
Macaulay from *The Amazing Brain*, by Robert Orenstein,
Richard Thompson, and David Macaulay. Copyright ©
1984 David A. Macaulay. Reprinted with permission of
Houghton Mifflin Company.)

neurons. These signals, in turn, are conveyed to the main body
of the nerve cell, where new electrical impulses are generated.
Outgoing impulses travel down a part of the cell called the
axon, whose endings, called *synaptic buttons*, are specialized
for the transmission of these impulses to other neurons. Axons
may be long or short, and may either end locally or travel to
other regions of the central nervous system and beyond. For
example, neurons whose cell bodies are up in the cerebral
cortex or brain stem may extend their long axons down into
the spinal cord. These axons join there with other nerve cells,
whose axons in turn travel out of the spinal cord to connect
with muscles and body organs.

The area of interface between two nerve cells is called a
synapse. In the following section, we will briefly describe the
events that occur at this junction, since an understanding of
the synapse is crucial in comprehending the effects of cocaine
on mood and behavior.

Events at the Nerve Cell Junction (Synapse)

The synapse plays a critical role in the central nervous system
because it is here where information is conveyed from one
nerve cell to another. In those few areas of the brain in which
nerve cells are extremely close together, synapses are *electro-
tonic*, which means that electrical impulses are transmitted
directly from neuron to neuron, much like an electrical current traveling down a connected wire. In the vast majority of
synapses, however, chemical substances called *neurotransmit-*

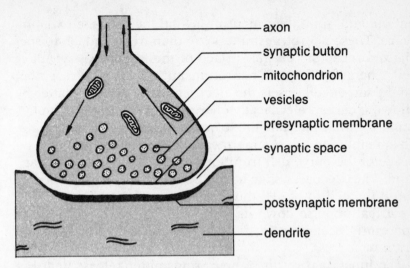

axon
synaptic button
mitochondrion
vesicles
presynaptic membrane
synaptic space

postsynaptic membrane
dendrite

Figure 2. Detailed diagram of a nerve synapse. (Illustration by David Macaulay from *The Amazing Brain*, by Robert Orenstein, Richard Thompson, and David Macaulay. Copyright © 1984 David A. Macaulay. Reprinted with permission of Houghton Mifflin Company.)

ters convey the electrical messages across the gaps that separate nerve cells.

A number of chemical compounds have been identified as neurotransmitters in the central nervous system. From the standpoint of our discussion of cocaine abuse, the most important of these are *norepinephrine* and *dopamine*. Like other transmitters, these compounds are stored in tiny sacs called *vesicles*, which are clustered in the synaptic button of the nerve cell (see Figure 2). In response to electrical changes on the surface of the nerve cell, these neurotransmitters are released into the synaptic space between neurons. By custom, the neuron that releases a neurotransmitter is designated as the *pre*synaptic neuron. The neuron that receives these transmitter molecules is designated as the *post*synaptic neuron. Almost every nerve cell functions as both a pre- and postsynaptic neuron, depending on its relationship to its neighboring nerve cells.

Transmission of an electrical impulse across the synapse occurs as follows. When the nerve impulse traveling down the axon reaches the synapse, the vesicles migrate to the end of the button and spill their neurotransmitters into the synaptic space. These neurotransmitters are then free to attach to specialized receptors on the surface of the target (postsynaptic) cell. The attachment of neurotransmitters to these receptors on the target cell upsets the electrical balance in the latter by allowing certain electrically charged ions like sodium, potassium, chloride, and calcium to cross the target cell membrane. This membrane is a semipermeable barrier that separates the inside of the nerve cell from the surrounding "extracellular" fluid. The electrical shift in the postsynaptic nerve cell may cause the cell to "fire," thus resulting in transmission of the electrical impulse down its own axon. This entire process is constantly occurring in neurons located in all areas of the brain.

The functional result of neurotransmitter release depends upon the effect each neurotransmitter has on its particular postsynaptic neuron. Some transmitters are *excitatory*, in that they facilitate transmission of an electrical impulse as described above. Other neurotransmitters are *inhibitory* in that their effect on postsynaptic nerve cells makes neuronal firing less likely. Since every nerve cell may receive either excitatory or inhibitory input from surrounding neurons, cell firing occurs only when the net accumulation of all of that cell's input reaches a threshold level.

The chemical reactions at the postsynaptic receptor are followed by release of the neurotransmitter compounds back into the synaptic space. There, these transmitters are either metabolized (broken down) by chemicals called *enzymes*, or they are returned into the presynaptic neuron to be broken down by enzymes inside the cell (see Figure 2), a process called *reuptake*. The most important of these enzymes is called *monoamine oxidase* (MAO).

Neurotransmitters are broken down into a variety of end products; recently developed laboratory techniques now enable us to measure these metabolic products in urine, blood, and cerebrospinal fluid. This ability, in turn, has allowed researchers to investigate the effects of drugs like cocaine on the production, release, and breakdown of various neurotransmitters. We can thus correlate drug-induced changes in mood and behavior with fluctuations in neurotransmitter activity. Experimental evidence to date suggests that cocaine, as well as other central nervous system stimulants, affects the levels of two and perhaps three known neurotransmitters in the brain. As research continues in this area, we may discover that other transmitter compounds are affected as well. For the purposes of this chapter, however, we will focus on the effects of cocaine on two compounds, norepinephrine and dopamine, which are thought to be important in the brain regulation of behavior, mood, level of consciousness, motor function, and hormonal output.

The Effects of Cocaine on Brain Function

Effects on Consciousness and Arousal

In both animals and humans, cocaine causes increased alertness and enhanced mental acuity when first administered, accompanied by marked changes in brain electrical activity. One area of the brain that is particularly affected by cocaine is the reticular formation, a nerve network running through portions of the brain stem that is thought to be involved in the regulation of consciousness, attention, and arousal.

The increased arousal and diminished need for sleep observed after cocaine use appears to be associated with the effects of the drug on certain central nervous system neurons that are thought to have an activating effect on human behavior. Cocaine appears to stimulate the release of norepinephrine and dopamine in these nerve cells; it also blocks the return (reuptake) of these transmitters from synaptic spaces back into presynaptic neurons, thus interfering with their metabolic breakdown. Both of these actions increase the availability of norepinephrine and dopamine in the synapse. Cocaine thus increases nerve cell firing in areas of the brain that control wakefulness and arousal.

Cocaine and the Perception of Pleasure

It is well established that cocaine functions as a powerful "reinforcer" in laboratory animals such as rats or monkeys. That is, once they have become acquainted with its euphoria-inducing effects, these animals will perform "work" such as repetitively pressing a lever to receive injections of cocaine. This finding is consistent with the drug's appeal in human beings, and the tendency of users to want to repeat the drug experience. Some researchers have speculated that this phenomenon is due to the effects of cocaine on certain "reward" areas of the brain, which are responsible for the perception of pleasure.

In an attempt to understand the brain mechanisms that underlie cocaine reinforcement, the drug has been given to cats, in which low doses will produce increased alertness, hyperactivity, and a desire to receive more cocaine injections. These effects can be diminished or entirely prevented by pretreating the animals with alpha-methylparatyrosine (AMPT), a drug that inhibits the production of both norepinephrine and dopamine. This finding suggests that one or both of these neurotransmitters is involved in the mediation of cocaine-seeking behavior. This hypothesis has been further tested in laboratory rats by administering drugs that destroy either norepinephrine-secreting or dopamine-secreting neurons, and then allowing the animals to self-administer intravenous cocaine. In one such study, destruction of those nerve pathways that use norepinephrine as a neurotransmitter failed to interfere with the reinforcing effects of cocaine. In other words, these animals continued to work for cocaine injections despite the lack of norepinephrine-mediated activity in their brains. In contrast, destruction of those neurons that used dopamine as a neurotransmitter resulted in a significant and long-lasting decrease in cocaine self-administration behavior.

These and other laboratory experiments have led to speculation that dopamine-containing neurons play an important role in mediating the positive reinforcing properties of cocaine. There is some evidence that opiate drugs also exert their reinforcing effects by activating dopamine-containing neurons in the brain, although opiates and cocaine apparently act at different locations in the brain and perhaps through different mechanisms.

The major site of action of cocaine on the dopamine system is in an area of the brain called the *nucleus accumbens*. Opiates probably act in an area called the *ventral tegmentum*, a part of the brain stem that contains the cells of origin of many dopamine-secreting neurons. In both instances, the primary reinforcing effects of these drugs is independent of their ability to induce physical dependence. Thus, the need in some users to repeat the drug experience over and over is caused more by the pursuit of euphoria than by a desire to ameliorate symptoms of drug withdrawal.

Stereotyped Behavior and Seizures

Although animals, like humans, vary in their responses to cocaine, a clear progression of dose-related effects may be observed during long-term cocaine use. Although low doses of cocaine produce hyperactivity, laboratory animals exposed to larger amounts of the drug begin to exhibit a peculiar form of compulsive stereotyped behavior. For example, cats receiving increasing doses of cocaine will repetitively sniff the same corner of a room for no apparent reason. Similar behavior is also seen in humans who have taken cocaine or other stimulant drugs over long periods of time. Some long-term users, for instance, may spend hours taking apart radios or television sets and putting them back together. Other similarly meaningless compulsive behaviors, particularly those requiring attention to detail, may also be observed in these individuals.

As in the case of hyperactivity, prior administration of alpha-methylparatyrosine (AMPT), a drug that inhibits the production of norepinephrine and dopamine, will prevent the development of stereotyped behavior in animals. This suggests that these neurotransmitters are involved in producing this compulsive behavior.

In rhesus monkeys, long-term administration of cocaine (such as over a six-month period) results in a progressive increase in pathological behavior, even in animals maintained on a fixed dose of the drug. Initially, the animals display the typical hyperactivity and stereotyped behavior observed in other species. After two months of cocaine use, however, they begin to demonstrate slowed movements, bizarre postures, staring, and a diminished ability to track objects in space. Some of these animals develop signs that suggest abnormalities in those nerve pathways that regulate voluntary and involuntary movement. Many also demonstrate an increased susceptibility to seizures, which is due to the tendency of cocaine to increase the electrical excitability of the brain. Indeed, there is evidence that prior to the onset of seizures in these animals, well-defined abnormalities of brain electrical activity may be observed, especially in an area of the brain known as the *limbic system*, which exerts substantial regulatory control over the emotions. These abnormal electrical discharges in the limbic system may also account for the behavioral changes observed during long-term, high-dose cocaine use in both animals and humans. Prior administration of drugs like carbamazepine (Tegretol), which lowers the level of electrical activity in the limbic system, will prevent the development of seizures and other types of abnormal behavior in these animals.

The Kindling Phenomenon

In studies of both animals and humans, long-term cocaine users appear to be more sensitive to the stimulatory effects of the drug than are novice or casual users. Thus, over time, long-term users may experience more excitatory effects from the same, or even smaller, doses of the drug.

In an attempt to explain the increasing sensitivity of long-term users to certain effects of cocaine, it has been postulated that repetitive experience with the drug may increasingly sensitize the brains of such individuals, a phenomenon known as *kindling*. Supporting this hypothesis are studies of laboratory animals in which neurons of the central nervous system that are repeatedly exposed to cocaine become sensitized to the effects of the drug and thus fire more readily with each succeeding drug exposure. During long-term use, these neurons fire even in response to relatively low doses of the drug. At the same time, one can detect abnormal electrical activity in the limbic systems of these laboratory animals, which can spread outside the emotional centers of the brain to cause generalized (grand mal) seizures.

In summary, long-term cocaine use appears to generate a form of pharmacological kindling that may account for the increased sensitivity of long-term users to the acute effects of the drug. Indeed, in some cases, the brain response to cocaine may be permanently altered. This would explain why, even after a long period of abstinence, individuals who had previously developed psychological difficulties as the result of long-term cocaine use may rapidly return to their cocaine-induced state even if exposed to extremely low doses of the drug.

Behavioral Effects of Long-Term Cocaine Use

Cocaine and Depression

Although cocaine initially produces euphoria, many otherwise normal users experience depression and anxiety after repeated high-dose use. These effects have also been noted during long-term use of other central nervous system stimulants like amphetamine or methylphenidate (Ritalin). Some long-term cocaine users simultaneously take central nervous system depressants (barbiturates, Valium, alcohol) or even opiates in an attempt to reduce their dysphoria and anxiety.

Research carried out by Dr. Robert Post and his colleagues at the National Institute of Mental Health provides further evidence that cocaine does not make everyone euphoric. Speculating that the drug may be an effective antidepressant, these investigators explored the effects of cocaine in clinically depressed patients. While some depressed individuals did experience a brief period of euphoria following intravenous cocaine use, others became more depressed. With continued use, particularly at high doses, the majority of these individuals became quite tearful, anxious, and distraught.

Depression ("crashing") following cessation of cocaine use is a fairly common phenomenon in both novice and experienced users. Although this may occur after brief usage of low doses of the drug, it is most common after stopping long-term high-dose cocaine use. New research by Drs. Frank Gawin and Herbert Kleber at Yale University School of Medicine has shown that crashing tends to occur in two phases. During the first one to three days of abstinence, users typically experience depression, irritability, anxiety, confusion, insomnia, and a gradually diminishing desire for more cocaine. This is followed by a one- to three-day period of depression, apathy, lethargy, increased appetite, and an enormous desire for sleep. Interestingly, this phase of the crash is often accompanied by an aversion to cocaine.

Following the initial crash, newly abstinent users typically spend one to five days in which they feel good, sleep normally, and experience little craving for cocaine because of their strong recognition of the drug's adverse effects. However, this period of calm may soon give way to another bout of depression, anxiety, irritability, lethargy, and severe boredom, frequently accompanied by a renewal of intense craving for cocaine. Over the next one to four days, bad memories about cocaine are gradually replaced by recollections of the drug's euphoric effects. Under these circumstances, if cocaine is available, relapse frequently occurs.

The biological mechanisms underlying the depression that results from cocaine withdrawal are also thought to be related to the effects of the drug on brain neurotransmitters, particularly norepinephrine. During prolonged cocaine use, brain neurons become depleted of these transmitters, as new production fails to keep up with the process of release and metabolic breakdown. As a result, a compound called 3-methoxy-4-hydroxyphenylglycol (MHPG), the major breakdown product of norepinephrine in the brain, is abnormally low during cocaine withdrawal, as it is in some patients with naturally occurring (rather than drug-induced) depression. In both instances, low levels of MHPG in urine, blood, or cerebrospinal fluid suggest that these individuals may be suffering from a deficiency of norepinephrine at functionally important receptor sites in the brain. Consistent with this hypothesis, the depressed mood that sometimes accompanies cocaine withdrawal can often be alleviated, although briefly, by taking yet another dose of cocaine, which releases whatever norepinephrine is still stored in individual brain neurons. At present, the role of dopamine and other neurotransmitters in cocaine-related depression remains unclear.

Cocaine Psychosis

Figure 3 shows the relationship between cocaine dosage, duration of use, and the development of cocaine-related psy-

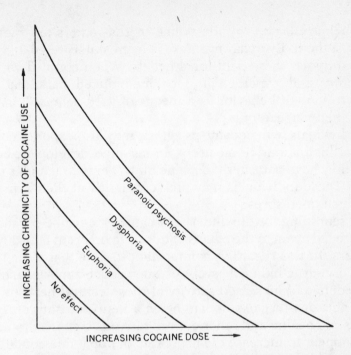

Figure 3. The interaction of dose and chronicity (length of use) in
determining the psychological reaction to cocaine. As the
dose or length of use increases, the reaction changes from
euphoria to dysphoria (feeling unwell or unhappy), and
eventually to paranoid psychosis. (Reprinted with permission from Post RM: Cocaine psychosis: a continuum
model. *American Journal of Psychiatry* 132:225–231, 1975.
Copyright © 1975 American Psychiatric Association.)

chopathology. As dose and duration of use increase, the cocaine-induced euphoria disappears and is replaced by depression, irritability, and—in some cases—psychosis.

The development of a psychotic state is more likely to occur
when high doses of cocaine are used over a long period of time.
However, a psychotic state can also occur suddenly in certain
vulnerable high-dose users. Cocaine psychosis is typically preceded by a transitional period that is characterized by increased suspiciousness, compulsive behavior, and dysphoric
mood. Users also become increasingly irritable, fault finding,
and eventually quite paranoid. Some psychotic individuals experience visual and/or auditory hallucinations, with persecu-
tory "voices" commonly heard. They may also feel that they

are being followed by the police or that others are plotting against them. Everyday events may be misinterpreted in a way that supports these delusional beliefs. When coupled with irritability and hyperactivity, cocaine-induced paranoia may lead to violent behavior as a means of "self-defense" against imagined persecutors.

Individuals with cocaine psychosis may also experience tactile hallucinations. Some users, for instance, develop the belief that they have parasites ("cocaine bugs") crawling under their skin. These individuals may pick constantly at their skin and produce open sores.

In searching for the underlying cause of cocaine psychosis, we are led again to the effects of this drug on brain neurotransmitters. In this regard, it is important to note that in patients with non-drug-induced psychosis, such as schizophrenia, there is evidence of increased activity of those central nervous system neurons that use dopamine as a neurotransmitter. High doses of cocaine and other central nervous system stimulants also appear to increase the firing rate of dopamine-containing neurons in the brain. During long-term cocaine use, for example, homovanillic acid, the major breakdown product of dopamine, is elevated in the cerebrospinal fluid of laboratory animals. This may be the result of cocaine-induced release of dopamine from presynaptic neurons or the drug's interference with the reuptake of this neurotransmitter into presynaptic neurons and its subsequent metabolic breakdown. Cocaine may also have a direct stimulatory effect on the dopamine receptors of postsynaptic neurons.

Regardless of the exact mechanism, long-term cocaine use appears to increase the activity of dopamine-containing neurons, and the development of stimulant-induced psychosis appears to be correlated with excessive levels of brain dopamine activity. Most researchers believe that this is also the underlying cause of the stereotyped behavior seen in both animals and humans after long-term cocaine use. Consistent with this hypothesis, the treatment of cocaine psychosis entails withdrawal of the drug and, in emergencies, the administration of psychoactive medications that block the effects of dopamine in postsynaptic neurons. Such drugs, called neuroleptics, are also effective in the treatment of schizophrenia and manic states, suggesting that increased brain dopamine may be an important factor in these conditions as well.

Adverse Reactions to Cocaine: Who Is Vulnerable?

Given the widespread popularity of cocaine and the tendency of many individuals to increase both their frequency of use and the dose consumed, one may wonder why the negative effects of the drug described in this chapter are not even more common. One explanation is that there are individual differences in the subjective response to cocaine, which are influenced by both genetic and environmental factors. In addition, the presence or absence of other psychological difficulties, the expectations of the user, and the setting in which the drug is used also influence the response to cocaine. Thus, individuals who are preoccupied by stressful life circumstances may be more vulnerable to the dysphoria and/or psychosis that sometimes accompany cocaine use. Relevant to this issue are the results of laboratory experiments in which administration of amphetamine, a related stimulant drug, to rats previously stressed by fighting or overcrowding appears to increase the likelihood of amphetamine overdose and death in these "stressed" animals.

Persons with overt or covert psychiatric disorders also appear to be more vulnerable to the disorganizing effects of cocaine, even after taking relatively low doses. For example, our research has shown that individuals suffering from chronic depression or manic-depressive illness run a particularly high risk of developing cocaine abuse problems. This may partly result from the powerful initial effect that cocaine has on some of these individuals, which encourages them to use the drug more frequently. Unfortunately, such persons may experience an exacerbation of their mental disorders as a result of their cocaine use. For example, Dr. Post's research (discussed earlier) showed that depressed patients are just as likely to experience dysphoria (feeling unwell or unhappy) as euphoria during early cocaine use, and they are more likely to experience depression as they increase their dose of the drug.

Individuals with underlying manic-depressive illness are also particularly sensitive to the effects of cocaine. Since cocaine increases the availability of both norepinephrine and dopamine in the brain, and since mania is thought to be a result, in part, of increased activity of these neurotransmitters, it is not surprising that manic states may be precipitated or exacerbated by cocaine use. Finally, persons with schizophrenia also appear to be more vulnerable to the disorganizing effects of cocaine. Indeed, they may manifest psychotic thinking or behavior even after relatively low doses of the drug.

Although we know that certain groups of individuals have a higher risk of developing cocaine abuse problems, there is no way to predict in advance who will, in fact, suffer adverse effects from the drug. It is precisely this unpredictability that makes cocaine use so hazardous. Cocaine is a very powerful drug that profoundly influences brain function. In the next chapter, we will discuss how these alterations of mood and behavior can lead to cocaine dependence.

5

Cocaine Dependence

During the worst New England snowstorm in nearly a century, Richard, a 25-year-old teacher, nearly froze to death because he had sold his car and his only winter coat for a quarter of an ounce of cocaine. Looking back on this decision was frightening, he said, "Because at the time, I made what seemed like the obvious choice. I just figured, 'Sell the coat, sell the car, get the coke.' I needed the cocaine more."

Eugene, a 41-year-old architect, related an angry conversation he had recently had with his wife:

> She had just caught me with cocaine again after I had managed to convince her that I hadn't used in over a month. Of course I had been tooting (snorting) almost every day, but I had managed to cover my tracks a little better than usual. So she said to me that I was going to have to make a choice—either cocaine or her. Before she finished the sentence, I knew what was coming, so I told her to think carefully about what she was going to say. It was clear to me that there wasn't a choice. I love my wife, but I'm not going to choose *anything* over cocaine. It's sick, but that's what things have come to. Nothing and nobody comes before my coke.

The World Health Organization (WHO) has defined drug dependence as "a state, psychic or also sometimes physical, resulting from the interaction between a living organism and a

55

drug, and characterized by behavioral and other responses that always include a compulsive desire or need to use the drug on a continuous basis in order to experience its effects and/or avoid the discomfort of its absence." The case examples described above highlight a central feature of cocaine dependence (we use the terms "dependence" and "addiction" interchangeably): both Richard and Eugene were preoccupied with cocaine. It had become their top priority—above physical well-being, above relationships, perhaps above basic survival instincts. These cases illustrate cocaine dependence in its most severe form, in which the individual thinks of little else but the drug, and cares neither for other people nor himself.

It is significant to note that the current WHO view of dependence (which is echoed in recent definitions by the National Institute on Drug Abuse and the American Psychiatric Association) does not distinguish between "physical" and "psychological" dependence. Indeed, the emphasis on the compulsion to use the drug repeatedly represents a departure from older definitions of drug dependence, which required the presence of tolerance (the need for markedly increased drug intake to achieve the desired effect) or of physical withdrawal symptoms. This redefinition of dependence was, in part, based on recent experience with cocaine. Since cocaine, unlike heroin or alcohol, does not cause a dramatic withdrawal syndrome, it was formerly considered "nonaddicting." This separation of physical versus psychological dependence was based on the mistaken belief that the avoidance of physical symptoms provides the primary motivation for drug users to continue their habit. Recent clinical experience and brain research (see Chapter 4) have shown otherwise: it is now widely accepted that cocaine can and does cause profound dependence, or addiction.

How does cocaine dependence develop? Who is at risk? In this chapter, we will attempt to answer these questions in several ways. First, we will describe a variety of theories that have been put forth to explain the etiology of dependence; we will then describe the typical course of cocaine dependence; finally, we will relate a case history of a young woman who developed profound dependence on cocaine after using the drug "safely" for several years.

Factors Contributing to Cocaine Dependence

Psychological Factors

One theory of cocaine dependence that is frequently espoused by health care professionals and addicts themselves is that cocaine abusers suffer from an underlying personality weakness, which is characterized by an inability to develop useful strategies for coping with stress. Other characteristics of this "addictive personality" include the tendency to be demanding, selfish, manipulative, and passive-aggressive. Addicts are often unable to tolerate even moderate amounts of frustration and frequently cannot understand or empathize with the feelings of others.

One major problem in accepting the validity of the concept of the "addictive personality" is the difficulty in determining the causes of these behaviors. Indeed, many of these traits may be the result of, rather than the cause of, drug use. For people who are forced to "hustle" on the street to support their continued use of an illegal drug, a certain degree of manipulativeness and selfishness may be necessary for their survival. These personality characteristics also reflect the power of addiction. As Richard and Eugene articulated so poignantly, the most significant relationship in the addict's life is with cocaine. If other relationships interfere with the ability to obtain or use cocaine, then those relationships will suffer. It is therefore easy to see how respect and empathy for others can also suffer.

Are manipulativeness, selfishness, and lack of empathy enduring personality traits in drug abusers, or are they the inevitable result of addiction? No one has clearly answered this question. However, similar personality descriptions have been applied to alcoholics, and a research project by scientists at Harvard Medical School helped to sort out some of the confusion surrounding the causes and consequences of that disorder. By studying a group of men from their adolescence into their mid-forties, Dr. George Vaillant and his colleagues were able to observe a subgroup of men who developed alcoholism. When the researchers reviewed the personality traits of the alcoholic subgroup that were recorded prior to the development of their alcoholism, they found that the personality characteristics frequently ascribed to these individuals—such as dependency, passive-aggressiveness, selfishness, and manipulativeness—were noted no more frequently in these individuals than in their nondrinking counterparts. The investigators therefore concluded that these personality traits (sometimes referred to as the "alcoholic personality") tend to occur as a *result* of long-term excess drinking, not as an underlying cause. Although the illicit nature of cocaine may create some differences between cocaine abusers and alcoholics, one could also hypothesize that cocaine abuse and alcoholism share a number of common features. It is therefore quite possible that a similar result would arise from an analogous study of cocaine abusers.

A second hypothesis, closely related to the "personality weakness" theory of cocaine abuse, is that some individuals abuse drugs in order to obtain relief from intolerable emotional states, particularly depression, anxiety, and anger. According to this "self-medication" hypothesis of cocaine use, an individual who is suffering from depression might seek out cocaine in order to relieve his low mood. In some instances, the initial use of cocaine to medicate these painful feelings is consciously planned by the user. In other instances, a serendipitous experience with the drug provides a deep sense of relief from emotional discomfort. In such cases, the individual may wish to repeat the comforting experience until a pattern of long-term use develops. We have performed research to test this self-medication hypothesis of cocaine abuse, and we have found a relatively high rate of mood disorders among long-term cocaine abusers admitted to our hospital unit. Approximately 20 percent of our cocaine abuse patients concurrently suffer from manic-depressive illness (recurrent mood swings shifting from euphoria to depression), and 15 percent have a serious depressive disorder.

One shortcoming of the "self-medication" theory of cocaine use is the fact that the drug's ability to relieve depression is generally short-lived. In a 1974 study at the National Institute of Mental Health, Dr. Robert Post led a team of researchers who tested the antidepressant effects of cocaine by giving the drug intravenously to a group of severely depressed patients. Dr. Post found that moderate doses of the drug caused temporary symptom relief in approximately one-third of the 23 patients studied. Another third of the patients felt little effect from the drug, and, interestingly, one-third of the patients experienced a worsening of their depression. When the drug was given in larger doses, only one of the eight depressed patients tested felt significantly better after being given cocaine. The rest either felt more depressed or experienced little effect from the drug. Thus, the study showed that there may be a subgroup of depressed patients who initially obtain temporary symptom relief from relatively small amounts of cocaine, thus accounting for the drug's appeal in these individuals. Prolonged high-dose use, however, may worsen depressive symptoms.

Dr. Post's study confirms the experience of many cocaine users who describe the drug more as a mood enhancer than a mood elevator. Many people use cocaine as a "party drug"; they find that cocaine initially heightens the experience of an already good mood. However, these same individuals generally avoid cocaine when they are depressed because they find that the drug worsens their already low mood.

Although cocaine initially causes euphoria in many occasional users, the majority of long-term cocaine abusers experience a mixture of depression, irritability, anxiety, and paranoia while on the drug. Despite these clearly noxious effects of chronic cocaine use on physical and psychological functioning, many long-term users continue to self-administer the drug until forced to discontinue it because of decreased drug availability, social or legal pressure, or medical complications. Clinicians who work with these patients are often at a loss to explain why they continue to use the drug despite its devastating consequences. Part of the explanation may rest in the difference between the actual drug experience and the individual's recollection of that experience. This discrepancy can in part be explained by the concept of *state-dependent learning*, in which events that occur during episodes of intoxication are poorly recalled once the individual is drug-free. Thus, cocaine addicts in drug treatment programs often recall with nostalgia even nightmarish episodes of intoxication.

State-dependent learning cannot, unfortunately, explain why some people feel compelled to continue using cocaine despite their recognition that it makes them feel worse than when they are drug-free. According to one patient,

I hate what the drug does. It makes me cry, it makes me crazy, it makes me think people are trying to kill me, it makes me turn all the lights off in my house and sit at my window for hours, just waiting for someone to climb down out of the trees so that I can get a gun and shoot him. I'm not like this usually. The drug does all of this to me. I hate what it does, but I love it. I love the looks of it, I love the taste, I love the smell, I love the feel, I love the action—I love it more than I've ever loved anything else in my life.

For such persons, continued cocaine use cannot be ascribed to the relief from unpleasant feelings, since these individuals often report feeling worse on drugs than off them. Some researchers have attempted to explain continued drug use in this group by suggesting that there are some cocaine abusers whose primary goal is to alter their mood, regardless of the direction of the change; they are simply looking for a new set of feelings. For some individuals who, for example, have suffered at the hands of abusive parents or who have been the victims of chaotic mood swings, the ability to control the timing of their mood changes may be so crucial that the type of mood change becomes comparatively unimportant.

Biological Factors

It has become increasingly apparent that understanding personality characteristics and inner psychological conflicts does not sufficiently explain the complexities of addictive behavior. Moreover, it is clear that individuals who experience significant psychological difficulties or social, cultural, or economic deprivation do not necessarily seek relief through the abuse of cocaine or other psychoactive drugs. Instead it appears that other factors place certain individuals at increased risk to develop drug problems.

Although research on the recent cocaine abuse epidemic is still in its infancy, much has been learned about the vulnerability to abuse other drugs and alcohol. One method of investigating the cause of substance abuse problems has been to study the families of drug-dependent patients and to design biological research projects to determine whether those who develop substance abuse problems are "biologically programmed" for dependence. For instance, some people may initially respond to these drugs in a particular way that increases the likelihood of future abuse problems. By examining findings from research that has already been done on other drugs and alcohol, perhaps we can hypothesize about some of the biological factors that may predispose certain individuals to abuse cocaine.

Family Studies. Although family studies of cocaine abusers and other drug-dependent individuals are rare, a great deal of informative research has been done on the families of alcoholics. It has long been recognized that alcoholism runs in families; the rate of alcoholism in first-degree relatives of alcoholics is approximately four times that of family members of nonalcoholics. Unfortunately, this finding does not tell us whether we are seeing the result of genetically inherited factors or of learned behavior. Brown hair runs in families; so does speaking English. However, the first trait is transmitted biologically, and the other is learned.

One could hypothesize that studying twins could help us to distinguish the varied contributions of "nature" and "nurture." The results of such studies support the presence of a genetically inherited vulnerability to the development of alcoholism; the rate of alcoholism in the identical twins of alcoholics is twice that of fraternal twins. These data suggest that there is probably a genetically inherited vulnerability to alcoholism that is shared more by identical twins, who have the same genetic endowment, than by fraternal twins, who have fewer genes in common. However, the fact that not all identical twins share alcoholism suggests that environmental factors also play a role. Indeed, it can be argued that identical twins often have a significantly different developmental experience from the general population as the result of being twins; this experience may adversely affect health and emotional well-being and promote the development of alcoholism.

Adoption studies, which compare the histories of biological and adoptive families of alcoholics who were adopted at birth, shed even more light on the relative contributions of genetic and environmental factors to the development of alcoholism. In these studies, the presence of alcoholism in a biological parent is the single most reliable predictor of alcoholism in the offspring, regardless of whether the child is adopted by alcoholics or nondrinkers. In contrast, adoptees born of nonalcoholic biological parents do not themselves develop alcoholism at any greater rate than the general population, even if they are reared by alcoholic adoptive parents. These studies lend considerable weight to the argument that genetic factors are important in the development of this disorder.

It may seem puzzling that a disorder like alcoholism, which involves voluntary behavior (drinking), can be genetically inherited. Several theories have been proposed to explain how this might be the case. Some have suggested that individuals vulnerable to the development of alcoholism may react to alcohol quite differently from those at less risk, even prior to the development of alcoholism. Some researchers have hypothesized that alcoholics have a dramatic response to their first exposure to drinking. However, research studies comparing the effect of alcohol on alcoholics versus nonalcoholics cannot differentiate whether the different responses in the two populations occur as the result of chronic alcoholism or whether the different response to alcohol was, indeed, a risk factor for the future development of alcoholism.

A University of California researcher, Dr. Mark Shuckit, developed an ingenious strategy to differentiate the causes of alcoholism from its effects. He studied a group of young men who were sons of alcoholics and compared them with men of the same age and educational background who had no family history of alcoholism. Because of their family backgrounds, the first group had a much higher risk for the future development of alcoholism, although none had current drinking problems. Dr. Shuckit felt that if he could detect differences between these two groups, then he might be able to identify risk factors that preceded alcoholic drinking. The results of the study were striking. Dr. Shuckit found that there were differences between the two groups, and that the sons of alcoholics exhibited a less dramatic response to alcohol than the sons of nonalcoholics. They were able to perform fine motor tasks more skillfully after drinking, and they felt less intoxicated than the sons of nonalcoholics.

Other comparative studies of these two groups have shown differences in certain blood hormone levels after drinking. Dr. Shuckit has hypothesized that the impaired ability of some drinkers to determine when they are becoming intoxicated may make it difficult for them to moderate their drinking. Conversely, others who are particularly sensitive to the effects of alcohol may alter their drinking patterns accordingly. For example, some Asians frequently experience flushing, rapid heart rate, abdominal pain, and weakness following relatively small doses of alcohol. These unpleasant effects, which may be caused by a relative lack of one of the enzymes that breaks down alcohol, have been cited as a major factor in the low rate of alcohol abuse in most Asian cultures.

Thus, we can see how the variability in the initial response to a drug may place some people at higher risk for future abuse problems. Although this hypothesis has been studied primarily in alcoholics, there is some evidence of a differential response to cocaine as well. In an experiment designed to assess the effect of cocaine on mood, Dr. Richard Resnick and his colleagues at New York Medical College administered 25 milligrams (approximately two lines) of cocaine to a group of regular users of the drug. Twelve subjects received the drug intravenously, and 12 received it intranasally. While most subjects experienced the drug as pleasant and relaxing, four of the intravenous users and two of the intranasal users reported dysphoric effects (feeling unwell or unhappy) after the period of euphoria. They described feelings of anxiety, fatigue, and depression and expressed a desire for more cocaine. One could hypothesize that individuals who experience the postcocaine "crash" more readily than other users may be at risk to develop cocaine abuse problems earlier than those who experience less craving for the drug after the euphoria ends.

Biological Markers in Addictive Disorders. Another line of inquiry in the search for the causes of addiction has been the attempt to find biological markers that may identify individuals who are at increased risk for the development of one or more of these addictive disorders. Biological markers may include abnormal physical characteristics or the degree of activity of particular chemicals in the body. Thus, for example (although the accumulated data are thus far inconclusive), there is some evidence that the level of activity of a chemical called *monoamine oxidase* (MAO), which can be measured in the blood, is decreased in alcoholics. Moreover, MAO levels appear to be reduced in the relatives of individuals with low MAO activity, particularly those relatives who are alcoholic themselves. As in the case of other biological markers, it is important to distinguish biological changes that precede and may predispose to the development of heavy drinking from those that may occur as a consequence of repetitive alcohol consumption.

Another group of biological markers that may affect the vulnerability to the subsequent development of drug and alcohol abuse involves the opiate-like compounds (*endorphins*) that are made in the body. These brain chemicals, which have been identified only in the last decade, appear to exert effects similar to opiate (narcotic) drugs. Thus, the release of endorphins after a minor injury will help a person to be less concerned about the pain he has just suffered. Some researchers have postulated that certain individuals are born with a deficiency of these substances, thus impairing their capacity to cope with physical or emotional distress. These persons may therefore be more likely to have a dramatic emotional response to opiate drugs such as morphine, heroin, or codeine. According to this theory, their use of opiate drugs fulfills a biological need and, in some respects, corrects a physiological abnormality.

Similar arguments have been advanced to explain the tendency among some people to abuse antianxiety drugs such as diazepam (Valium). These individuals may be congenitally deficient in certain naturally occurring antianxiety compounds, thus theoretically rendering them less able to handle "normal" amounts of anxiety. Using the same reasoning, some investigators have suggested that abusers of central nervous system stimulants like cocaine, which increase turnover of brain chemicals called *catecholamines*, particularly norepinephrine and dopamine (see Chapter 4), may be suffering from an underlying deficiency of catecholamines in their brains, which is at least temporarily relieved by self-administration of these compounds. This relatively low level of brain catecholamines may show up as symptoms of depression.

Social Factors

Although recent advances in pharmacology and brain chemistry have helped to elucidate the mechanism of action of co-

caine, biological factors alone cannot explain a behavioral phenomenon as complicated as addiction. It is important to keep
in mind that drug abuse occurs within a social context. Thus,
the environment in which drug-taking occurs profoundly influences the nature of the user's behavior. Critical environmental
influences include relationships with family, friends, and
peers, as well as the individual's role within larger social insti-
tutions, including religion, social class, and the legal system.

Drugs as a Social Lubricant. A number of drug users recount
that their initial experiences with drugs like cocaine, alcohol,
and marijuana were designed to help them communicate better with others. Indeed, in small quantities these substances
decrease inhibitions and at times enable people to express
feelings that they would ordinarily keep to themselves. However, with heavier use of these drugs, their facilitating effect on
interpersonal communication is lost; people highly intoxicated
on marijuana tend to become self-absorbed and somnolent,
while large amounts of cocaine or alcohol may cause increased aggressiveness and poor judgment.

From the standpoint of peer group interaction, drug use may
provide the focus for shared activity. A number of research
studies have shown that people who use large amounts of
drugs or alcohol tend to cultivate relationships with other
heavy drug users. These individuals, who often have little sense
of their own identity, find within the drug-using peer group a
degree of acceptance, a clear set of behavioral expectations,
and approval for continuing their drug-using life-style. Adolescents appear to be particularly vulnerable to this subtle form of
peer pressure.

As an extension of peer group approval of substance abuse,
we have witnessed several periods in history during which
drug use was the behavioral expression of certain social and
cultural values. Thus, during the 1960s, the use of LSD and
other hallucinogens took place in the context of a rebellion
against traditional middle class values. The phrase "turn on,
tune in, and drop out" suggested that hallucinogen use was one
means by which certain groups could separate themselves
from what they saw as an unjust society.

Cocaine use today often occurs as an expression of financial and social success—of having "made it." According to Paul, a 28-year-old stockbroker,

> Doing coke alone defeats part of the purpose of it. You do it around certain people to show who you are. You're up and coming, you're one step ahead of the game, and they'd better watch out. People used to join country clubs as a status symbol so that they could talk about it to their friends and co-workers. In our office, people invest in "blow" for the same reason. Unfortunately, it's a damned expensive and damaging way to give people the message that you're hot.

Finally, some individuals become involved with illicit drug use because they are attracted to the deviant life-style that often accompanies such use. For them, the excitement of the illegal activity that is often required to obtain drugs may be as rewarding as the pharmacological effects of the drugs themselves. Others may find that the use of these drugs may facilitate risk taking or engaging in deviant behavior that they have learned to enjoy.

> A 22-year-old man who had a history of rebellious behavior both within his family and at school left his small midwestern hometown in order to go to New York, where his stated goal was to become a heroin addict. "I wanted to get addicted to heroin because I could think of no other behavior which was more proscribed by society." He said that for the initial several months, he did not particularly enjoy the pharmacological experience of intoxication. However, he relished the challenge of stealing in order to pay for his habit and enjoyed mingling with "the netherworld of our society." He eventually became strongly addicted to heroin and cocaine.

Familial Factors. Many clinicians and researchers have attempted to determine the possible role of family relationships in the development of substance abuse. For example, it has been noted that although drug abusers often pursue a life-style that most people would term deviant, they frequently remain involved and perhaps overly entangled with their families of origin. A recent study of heroin addicts, for instance, revealed that 59 percent of those studied still lived with their mothers or a female blood relative at age 30. Numerous authors have attempted to describe family backgrounds that might predispose children to drug dependence. One of the most frequently described patterns is a combination of overindulgence and overly harsh, arbitrary punishment. These may both be seen in one parent or may reflect a difference between the mother and father. The overprotectiveness may deprive children of experiencing the normal anxieties and frustrations of growing up. Such individuals may therefore be at an increased risk to seek pharmacological relief from unpleasant feelings because of a lack of other coping skills. The harshness of discipline may allow children to be similarly harsh on others in an attempt to rationalize some of the antisocial acts that often accompany drug addiction.

Although such theories of addiction are interesting and at times useful, they have never stood the test of rigorous study. There are clearly many individuals raised within similar family constellations who never develop drug problems. Indeed, many substance abusers have siblings who do not have similar difficulties. Thus, merely invoking pathogenic family interactions cannot explain the development of substance abuse disorders. No scientific research has ever demonstrated a correlation between any particular family setting or early childhood experience with the subsequent development of alcohol or drug abuse. Moreover, the clinical experience of those who work with many substance abusers and their families reveals much more about their diversity than their similarity.

Sociocultural Factors. We have seen the ways in which psychological, biological, and family experiences can influence an individual's drug choice and his subsequent pattern of drug use. The social, cultural, religious, and legal values of one's larger society also profoundly affect the use of drugs and alcohol. For example, the Harrison Narcotics Act of 1914, which outlawed cocaine, nearly wiped out the use of a drug that had been enormously popular in America during the previous 25 years. The recent growth of cocaine use in this country has in large part been related to the prestige that has been conferred on the drug by certain segments of our society. There are some social groups for whom the use of cocaine is so commonplace that abstaining may raise eyebrows. According to a 36-year-old advertising executive,

Where I work, people use coke like most people use coffee. It's just a given that you do some "toot" just about every day. Maybe it's part of the creative process. It's as if everyone around you is so up that if you're not using coke, you're going to fall behind. In our office, if you don't do toot, most people are going to think you're an addict who's trying to quit. Everyone around here can afford to buy coke pretty regularly, so what other reason could you have to not use it?

The influence of social setting and peer group acceptance on drug-using behavior is not limited to cocaine. Indeed, the influence of these factors on patterns of drug use was never more powerfully demonstrated than during the Vietnam War, in which it was estimated that one-third of all American combat soldiers between the ages of 17 and 23 used opiates, and in particular heroin. Approximately half of this group used these drugs regularly. It appears that several factors contributed to this epidemic of heroin use. First, the drugs were easily available; high-quality heroin could be traded for several packs of American cigarettes. In addition, heroin could be used without involving street crime, dirty needles (many people used the drug intranasally), and high-priced drug dealers. Finally, the shared horror of the Vietnam experience among combat troops led to widespread acceptance within that group of pharmacological self-treatment for anxiety, depression, paranoia, rage, and despair.

The use of heroin among such a large number of American soldiers in Vietnam illustrates a well-recognized trend in the epidemiology of drug abuse—that psychopathology becomes a less important risk factor for the use of a given drug when the use of that drug becomes more normal and accepted within the society. In other words, the use of heroin in Vietnam was not restricted to a few individuals with long-standing emotional disorders. Rather, the combination of drug availability and a high degree of stress led a large number of people who would not ordinarily use heroin to do so. This phenomenon was corroborated by follow-up studies of opiate-dependent troops, showing that less than 10 percent of that group ever used opiates again after returning to the United States. Moreover, less than 2 percent of soldiers who were opiate-dependent in Vietnam continued to have serious opiate-related problems after their return from Southeast Asia.

These results are markedly different from studies of individuals who become addicted to heroin in their home environment. Many of the latter group experience cycles of addiction, detoxification, and subsequent relapse that often stretch over a period of years. Therefore, the setting in which drug use and addiction occur, drug availability, and the shared values of one's peer group all play important roles in determining the future outcome of an individual's drug use.

Unfortunately, the availability of cocaine continues to climb, worldwide production of the drug continues to increase, prices are falling, and the purity of street cocaine is rising. In addition, cocaine is still viewed by many people as a relatively harmless, highly valued celebration drug. This combination of factors has allowed an increasing number of people to be exposed to cocaine. As we have seen, increased exposure leads to more cocaine addiction.

Religious and cultural mores may also have a powerful influence on the use of drugs or alcohol in a society. Epidemiologic studies, for example, have shown that certain ethnic or religious groups (such as Irish Americans and American Indians) have greater than average rates of alcoholism, while others (such as Asians and Jews) have relatively fewer alcoholics. Several sociocultural factors have been identified as being potentially important influences on drinking patterns within a society. Among those factors that are felt to correlate with a relatively low rate of alcoholism are 1) drinking with people of the opposite sex, 2) drinking across generational lines (grandparents, parents, and children drinking together), 3) drinking with meals, 4) drinking as part of a religious ceremony or holiday celebration, and 5) belonging to an ethnic, religious, or social group that considers drunkenness to be a disgrace. Although it is difficult to draw an exact parallel with cocaine, we can see how a wide range of social values exert their influence on the individual's of drugs and alcohol.

Behavioral Factors

Another helpful perspective in our understanding of addiction is that of learning theory. Two key concepts that represent the cornerstones of learning theory include *operant reinforce-*

ment and *classical conditioning.* Operant reinforcement refers to the ability of a particular event or response within the environment to increase the frequency of a specific behavior. A simple example can be seen in training animals. If you wish to teach an animal a particular piece of behavior, then you will reward it with food, affection, or some other positive action when it performs that behavior. If the animal continues to perform the desired behavior because it has been given the reward, then the reward is said to be reinforcing. Using this principle, scientists have found that animals can be taught to perform "work," usually in the form of repeatedly pressing a lever, in order to receive injections of certain psychoactive drugs, including cocaine. Over time, the animal may be required to work harder and harder in order to continue receiving the drug.

These types of experiments give us a rough approximation of the relative reinforcing properties of various psychoactive drugs. Not surprisingly, animals have been enticed in such experiments to work for opiates, amphetamine, nicotine, barbiturates, phencyclidine (PCP), and alcohol. However, their response to cocaine was dramatic and unparalleled. Under conditions of unlimited access to intravenous cocaine, rhesus monkeys continued to work for cocaine and self-administer the drug until it caused their death.

Some behavioral scientists believe that the powerful reinforcing property of cocaine is sufficient to explain continued drug-seeking behavior even in the absence of preexisting psychological problems, poor interpersonal relationships, biological vulnerability, or peer group pressure. These scientists believe that cocaine is such a powerful drug that it can lead to severe addiction in virtually anyone, as long as it is easily available. This belief has led some outspoken advocates of the legalization of marijuana and heroin to express some misgivings about the legalization of cocaine, since it appears that the growing availability of the drug and the concurrent drop in price has led to a large increase in the number of cocaine-related problems in this country.

Classical Conditioning and Craving. Classical conditioning was first described at the turn of the century by Russian psychologist Ivan Pavlov, who reported this phenomenon after performing experiments with his dog. Pavlov found that when he repeatedly rang a bell while presenting his dog with food, the dog would salivate at the sound of the bell, because it was concurrently receiving food. When Pavlov later rang the bell without presenting the food, the dog continued to salivate because it had mentally paired the bell with the food to such an extent that the ringing of the bell continued to evoke this *conditioned response*. The concept of Pavlovian (classical) conditioning is important in understanding *craving*, which can be defined simply as a strong desire for drugs.

Craving may show itself primarily as an emotional state, or it may be accompanied by physical symptoms. The desire for drugs tends to increase when drugs are available and diminish when they are not easily attainable. Craving is often stimulated by conditions previously associated with drug-taking activity; these may include psychological or interpersonal stress, being in the presence of former drug-using companions, or entering a neighborhood in which one has previously taken drugs. Increased craving in response to feelings, places, or people associated with previous drug experiences is another example of a classically conditioned response. This type of reaction may at times trigger relapse.

> A 30-year-old man was hospitalized for a month because of long-term cocaine abuse. During that time, he engaged in individual psychotherapy, became involved in Narcotics Anonymous, and attended several groups daily, most of them focusing on ways in which cocaine had adversely affected his life. Two days after being discharged to home, he received a telephone call from his drug dealer, who said, "Where have you been? I've been holding an ounce of cocaine for you for weeks." The patient replied, "Great! When can we get together?" He relapsed that day, but later stated emphatically that he had had no desire to take cocaine before talking with his dealer.

This vignette clearly illustrates the powers of classical conditioning; under conditions of high drug availability, intense craving can be quickly stimulated and may trigger conditioned behavior in an almost automatic way. Under these circumstances, a cocaine abuser can quickly lose sight of the potentially harmful consequences of his actions. Because of such behavioral responses, we recommend that individuals who are trying to stop cocaine avoid former drug-using companions and localities.

Conditioned responses may include physiological changes in addition to psychological reactions. For example, rats that have been previously addicted to opiates will demonstrate signs of withdrawal when placed in an environment in which they have undergone withdrawal in the past. This phenomenon of "conditioned withdrawal" has been observed in humans as well.

> A 29-year-old man was hospitalized for the treatment of heroin addiction. After four weeks of treatment, he returned to his former job, which required him to ride the subway past the stop at which he had previously bought his drugs. Each day, when the subway doors opened at this location, the patient experienced enormous craving for heroin, accompanied by tearing, a runny nose, abdominal cramps, and gooseflesh. After the doors closed, his symptoms disappeared, and he went on to work.

This young man experienced symptoms of heroin withdrawal in this locale when the doors were open because this represented a period of high drug availability. In his mind, heroin withdrawal and this particular subway station were as clearly paired as were the bell and food for Pavlov's dog. Thus, he experienced increased drug craving in the most hazardous of all circumstances: when drugs were readily available.

Many substance abusers find that as their addiction develops, they become "hooked" on conditioned stimuli: drug paraphernalia, needles, razor blades, mirrors, "coke spoons," stealing, scheming, and procuring drugs. For some users, these components of the addictive life-style become as important as the pharmacological activity of the drugs. Thus, there are some individuals, known as "needle freaks," who will inject themselves with water if there are no drugs available, because they derive pleasure merely from the experience of injection itself. When these conditioned stimuli constitute an important part of an individual's addiction, altering the pattern of drug dependence can be very difficult without making major changes in life-style at the same time.

The Course of Cocaine Dependence

Not all cocaine users develop dependence. Rather, the use of cocaine occurs along a continuum from one-time experimentation to severe addiction. Cocaine use causes very few problems for some individuals, creates temporary difficulties in others, and ruins or ends the lives of still others. This unpredictability is one of the most dangerous properties of cocaine. Certain drugs, such as heroin, have acquired a dangerous reputation that frightens away many potential users. Many people who are afraid of heroin are willing to experiment with cocaine, however, since they perceive it as a "soft" drug.

Dr. Robert L. DuPont, former director of the National Institute on Drug Abuse, has called Experimentation and First Time Use the first of four stages of the drug dependence syndrome, with the latter three stages being Occasional Use, Regular Use, and Dependence. Experimentation with cocaine is often disappointing; many first-time users wonder why cocaine is so popular, and they frequently feel that the drug is overrated and overpriced. Some users will stop at this stage simply because they had only wanted to try the drug once; others will cease cocaine use because of their disappointment in its effects. Some who have had an unremarkable experience, however, will be convinced by their friends to try the drug several more times in order to get used to it. Many patients have told us that they did not truly enjoy cocaine until they had used it sporadically for weeks or even months. Some of these individuals had incorrectly believed that their initial lack of response to cocaine would protect them against future difficulties with the drug. Unfortunately, they were mistaken, since the course of cocaine dependence is highly variable. Although some people realize soon after exposure to cocaine that they cannot stop using the drug, others may use cocaine with few adverse consequences for months or years before they become dependent.

Unlike the group mentioned above, there is a small but significant group of individuals who are profoundly affected by their first dose of cocaine; some develop a craving for the drug after using the drug just once. A 37-year-old man described such an experience as follows:

I was at a party with a group of friends, and at 11 o'clock, this guy brings out some cocaine. I had never seen the stuff before, and I had never been much of a drug user. Maybe I'd smoked a few joints here and there, but nothing serious. I never even drank heavily. But I was having a good time and was feeling rather adventurous that night, so I decided that I would try some coke. A bunch of us sat around and snorted the stuff, and after two little lines of this drug, it was all over. I've never felt anything like it in my life. From that moment on, I knew that cocaine was the drug for me. It was as if I had been born to use cocaine. I felt that I could talk to people, like I was the life of the party, that I could think more clearly, that I was in control. In one minute, I went from being an ordinary, shy, straight-arrow guy to being a king. So far, so good. The problem started a couple of hours later, when the party broke up. Everybody else went home smiling and talking about what a great time they had had. All I could think about was how to find more cocaine. I swear, in two hours I was well on my way to becoming an addict.

Although this man's story is dramatic and unusual, it is not unique. The progression from experimentation to dependence can take place over an extended period of time or, as in the case cited above, may occur quite quickly. For this man and others like him who have a dramatic response to cocaine, dependence is not a foregone conclusion. Some people are frightened by their dramatic reaction to the drug and therefore avoid it, lest they become dependent. Others continue to use the drug on occasion, without progressing to further stages of cocaine abuse, because they set strict guidelines for their drug use and never violate them. However, it is quite important to realize that the progression of drug addiction is typically filled with broken promises that are made to oneself, friends, and family members.

How Dependence Develops

Dependence on cocaine may occur under a variety of circumstances and may develop in a matter of days or over a period of several years. However, there are certain aspects of the addictive process that are nearly universal. One major feature of the disorder is the continued use of the drug despite its adverse consequences. Many people in our society develop *temporary* problems as a result of alcohol or drug use. However, the majority of people who have such reactions alter their future behavior to avoid experiencing the problem again. Thus, an individual who realizes that he is intoxicated when driving home from a restaurant may refrain from drinking and driving in the future. An addict, however, does not react in this way, because he typically fails to see the connection between his drug use and his difficulties.

This inability to appreciate the destructive effects of drug use is generally referred to as *denial.* Indeed, addiction has often been called "a disease of denial." Denial becomes an essential part of the addictive process because most addicts care more about their drugs than about anything or anyone else in their lives. The first goal of any addict is obtaining and using drugs; everything else on the addict's list of priorities is tied for a distant second. Relationships, work, money, and physical health become secondary considerations.

Addiction changes one's values, so that things that were formerly important no longer seem to matter. This was demonstrated quite dramatically in the case of a 29-year-old cocaine abuser referred to one of us (Dr. Weiss) for a consultation.

Doctor: How much cocaine do you use in a week?
Patient: About three grams.
Doctor: So you're spending about $300 a week. How much money do you take home from work?
Patient: Maybe $350.
Doctor: That doesn't leave you much money for anything else.
Patient: That's right.
Doctor: What do you do for rent and food money?
Patient: I eat enough to get by, but I'm probably going to be evicted soon, since I can't pay the rent.
Doctor: So you spend your rent money on cocaine?
Patient: I keep telling myself when I get my paycheck that I'm going to drive directly to my landlord's place and pay him off. The problem is that I always make a little coke stop on the way, and I don't have any money by the time I get to my landlord's place. I keep telling myself that something will work out, but I'm not sure how.

This patient is caught in the throes of cocaine addiction; his values have been altered so severely that the acquisition of cocaine has assumed greater importance in his life than food and shelter. When drugs become this important to an individual, then he physically and psychologically protects himself against anything that might interfere with the continuation of his drug use. For the addict, this generally means protecting himself vigilantly against facing reality, for heavy drug use invariably causes problems. Through the use of denial and rationalization, the addict can blame his problems on other people, on bad luck, and on anyone or anything *except* his drug use.

Fortunately, repeated confrontation with reality may interfere with the denial process, and many long-term cocaine abusers eventually come to realize the damage that the drug is causing them. However, even those addicts whose denial breaks down may have difficulty stopping the drug. If a heavy user makes a sincere but unsuccessful effort to stop using cocaine, panic may set in. A 26-year-old salesman described this phenomenon:

> For months, people have been telling me that my cocaine use was a problem, that I was ruining my wife's life, that I was ruining my son's life, and that I needed to stop using the drug. Of course, I thought everybody was crazy. Even though my life got a little weird every once in a while, I thought things were basically under control. I also sincerely felt for a long time that I could stop using the drug anytime I set my mind to it. My wife constantly gave me grief about it, so I decided that to save the marriage I would really give it a try. I decided on New Year's Day that I was going to stop using cocaine. On January 4th, I started using the drug again. At that point, I knew I was in trouble—deep trouble. I felt that I had no way out, and that I was never going to be able to stop using this drug. Here I was, this hotshot salesman, and I truly believed that I was going to die a drug addict. I was so scared that I couldn't think straight. The only thing I knew was that I had to hide my cocaine use from my wife. I felt so guilty and hopeless, all I could do was use more and more cocaine to try not to think about it. Never in my life have I felt such constant anxiety and despair. I knew that if I didn't get myself into a treatment program in a hurry, I would kill myself. I felt that hopeless.

This man's poignant account describes the desperation of the addict, the guilt that often ensues, and the inability to use that guilt in a constructive manner to alter behavior. Rather than stopping the cocaine use to lessen his guilt, the addict's sense of powerlessness over his addiction leads him to use even more heavily in order to escape his guilty feelings.

Thus, we often see a progression from the initial euphoria of cocaine use to a stage of temporary drug-related difficulties; these problems may lead to either a reduction of or complete end to cocaine use, or to denial of the true cause of the difficulties. If the latter occurs, the drug-related problems may become more intense and frequent; this may eventually lead to a reduction in the level of denial, although it may be too late at this point to easily turn the drug problem around. Some individuals will still be able to stop at this point, while others will attempt to stop drug use and fail. These individuals often enter a period of rapidly increasing drug use, borne out of panic, desperation, hopelessness, and a feverish attempt to dispel these feelings.

Understanding Denial

In describing the course of addiction, we stressed the central importance of *denial* in the worsening of the disorder. What exactly do we mean by this term? More importantly, how can we understand it? Many family members, friends, colleagues, and health care professionals working with substance abusers have been amazed at the capacity of these individuals to seemingly ignore the role of their drug taking in the creation of their difficulties. Bill, a 34-year-old cocaine addict who had been drug-free for three years, explained his own denial quite well.

I had been an occasional coke user, maybe once or twice a month, for a couple of years before I started to get into it pretty heavily. I had just started making some money with a business that I owned, and I was running in some pretty fast circles. Offering cocaine was just a way of saying hello to some of those people. Deep in my heart, I knew I had a problem a few months later when I realized that my new-found money and a lot of my savings were all going for drugs.

For example, there was the day when I went out to buy my two-year-old son a birthday present, and I came home with an empty pocket and a sore nose. My wife confronted me, and I made this grandstand play. I took out two Bibles that we had in the house and put my right hand on them and swore to God that I had not been using cocaine. I made up this elaborate story about having been unable to find our son the perfect present, and I said that I would go out the next day to another store to find it. As I was telling this story, I knew perfectly well that I was lying, but it seemed to make sense. In that particular frame of mind, I hadn't done anything wrong. I was still high, and the drug reinforced my denial, because it made me feel so good. I felt that this drug was saying to me, "The hell with her, Bill. Just get her off your back. I can make you feel better."

At that point, I truly believed that I needed the drug more than anything else in the world. I was reacting as if I had a life-threatening illness and that the cure for it was to take as much cocaine as I could get, as often as possible. With that as my assumption, lying meant nothing to me, people meant nothing to me, my work meant nothing to me, my beautiful little boy meant nothing to me. What I didn't realize at the time—but what is perfectly clear to me now—is that I did have an illness. But the illness was caused by cocaine, rather than being cured by it. I think that I was denying the reality of what was going on because I felt so bad without cocaine, and because I felt so powerless over that drug, that I couldn't bear thinking about life without it. I had to try to convince myself that cocaine was not my problem, because admitting the truth would force me to either accept being an addict or try to give up the drug. Both choices were totally intolerable.

As illustrated in Bill's story, the progression of addiction is generally accompanied by a gradual alteration of a person's expectations of himself in order to fit his behavior. This process occurs in all of us at times, and it can be quite adaptive, such as during aging. As we grow older, we realize that we are physically less able to perform certain feats that we used to be able to accomplish during our youth. It is a sign of maturity to accept this fact and to change our expectations of ourselves accordingly. This same phenomenon also occurs in addicts, but it occurs in response to their addictive disorder instead of as the result of normal development. As their behavior—lying, stealing, or cheating—deviates from their former goals for themselves, their expectations change; they may rationalize these acts as if they are an unavoidable by-product of their hostile environment. Frequently, the first step in recovery from cocaine abuse is the acceptance that this type of behavior is not necessary, but is a symptom of an illness.

The following interview illustrates the use of denial in a 48-year-old executive, who was brought by his wife to see one of us (Dr. Weiss) for a consultation. Mr. A's wife had complained that he was jeopardizing his formerly successful business with erratic decisions and poor management skills; he was irritable

usually buy a quarter of a gram for $25, or I'd split a half gram with a girlfriend or two. A quarter of a gram was only good for about 10 lines, but it would last me a weekend. I'd go out on a Friday night, do two lines and leave the rest in my apartment, go to a club, have a few drinks, party, hang out, go back to my apartment, wake up on a Saturday morning and maybe do a line, go to the beach all day if it was summertime, and then come back and do the rest of the coke on Saturday night before I went out.

I can't say the drug hurt my love life at that point. Hell, I had good sex when I did coke. I liked it. Not only that, but a lot of times I'd see a guy I wanted to meet. If I had a half gram of coke, I could have him in my apartment with me just like that. I mean, I'd go to a club, and I'd be a little bit buzzed, and I'd have a half gram of coke with me and I'd see a really good looking guy and I'd just walk up to him because I was Superwoman. Since I had already done a few lines, I was high enough to believe that no one was going to reject me. If anyone did, I'd think, "Well, the hell with you, I don't want you anyway." All that was rationalizing. So I would just walk up to a guy, and I would say, "Hi, do you want to do some lines?" It was just an easy way to meet somebody, not only sexually, but just if I didn't want to be alone. If you have drugs, especially coke, anybody will be with you.

Problem Use

As time went on, I started using cocaine in the morning, before work, during breaks at work, and sometimes right in the middle of my office if I was alone for a few minutes. I thought that was cool because I didn't get caught. Also when I did coke I felt the euphoria that told me I would never get caught.

The first behavior that should have signalled to me that I was in trouble came when I started selling my jewelry. I wasn't making a lot of money, and I couldn't afford to buy coke because by this time I was going through half a gram on the weekends. Sometimes I'd even use half a gram on the weekend and a quarter of a gram during the week. So, piece by piece, I started selling my jewelry. My grandfather had been a fine jewelry maker, and he had given me this beautiful collection of

rings, necklaces, and bracelets that had always had tremendous sentimental value to me. I knew when I was selling it that
I was never going to get it back, but I thought that having one
less ring wasn't as important as having more friends. Now I was
attracting false "friends" from turning people on, and these
people weren't going to come around me if I didn't have any
drugs. So I said to myself, "I have lots of jewelry. I'm not going
to miss one piece, and I'm going to have friends all weekend
long." Then I sold the next one and then the next one and I
kept telling myself the same thing. When I sold my first piece of
jewelry, I was probably spending $80 a week on cocaine for
myself, and I was turning a lot of other people on. But I swear,
at that time, I didn't think anything was wrong. I thought that
was just the way it was supposed to be.

My performance at my job was going straight downhill; I'd
be up till four or five o'clock in the morning snorting coke, and
maybe by six o'clock my heart would stop pounding and I
could fall asleep. When all the "normal" people were getting
up to go to work, I was sleeping off the drug high from the night
before. So I missed a lot of work. But in my head, I said to
myself, well, you're new at this job, and you're living down-
town, where there's a lot of things to do besides work. I really
thought that this was all happening just because I was in a new
job, and that once I got used to it, I'd get into a healthy pattern
and everything would all be okay.

It was around this time that the lying and manipulating
started, too. One day, my mother asked me why I never wore
my jewelry anymore. I had to lie. I told her that someone had
broken into my apartment. I said, "Ma, I came home one day
and a necklace was gone; you know the creeps that live in the
city." The incredible thing was that the story came out so easily,
so naturally, I think I believed it myself. I know now that I was
using denial pure and simple, and that I blamed my problems
on everything and everyone except for myself and cocaine. I
was able to deceive myself so easily because I felt that I had to
have the drug. I think that cocaine itself also gave me false
feelings. I was starting to do coke every day at this point, Monday through Friday, a line here, a line there, and then 10 or 15
lines, sometimes 20 lines on the weekend. I think that the
cocaine along with the pot and the alcohol, which "evened me

out," gave me false feelings. When I got high, I always felt that I was okay, that there was nothing to worry about.

Addiction

I'd now reached a point where I didn't have many options if I wanted to keep using coke: I could deal, I could steal, or I could sell myself. Before I was through, I did all three. I started with dealing. One of the guys who sold me coke was a big time Valium dealer, and he wanted someone else to make his deliveries for him. I knew that I looked innocent enough, so I figured that the odds of my getting arrested were pretty low. And I couldn't argue with the pay: a half gram of coke per delivery. So I thought I was on top of the world. I was making an average of two deliveries a day and snorting a gram of coke every day without spending a penny. The dealing also gave me a sense of power. People needed me to get their high. If someone was really wasted on coke and he wanted to come down with Valium, he had to rely on me. It was as if I was controlling everything that was going on.

As that year went on, I started dealing coke, too, at first for this guy, then for myself. He would give me an eighth of an ounce [just over 3 grams], and I would take it back to my apartment and lock the door, because the coke was starting to make me paranoid at this point. Then I'd try a line to figure out how good it was. Even though I wasn't an expert, I thought I was. Depending on how pure I thought the coke was, I would cut it. A lot of times, especially toward the end of that year, I would keep half for myself, cut the other half, and sell it. I'd give him the money for the eighth of an ounce and I'd get a free gram and a half. That, of course, would be gone in about two hours. I was using two or three grams each weekend night, and about a gram and a half every weeknight. At this point, I never missed a night. And I could keep on working because I had access to enough Valium to get to sleep every night; usually two or three pills would do the trick.

As far as I was concerned, all of this was great. Then one morning, at about eight o'clock, after having slept for only about one hour, this guy that I was in partnership with knocked at my door, and he was out of his mind. I didn't know what was wrong with him. He came into my apartment, ripped it apart, and beat me up. He cracked a glass jar over my head, punched me in the face, and I didn't know why he was flipping out. I found out the next day that he was freebasing [smoking freebase cocaine; see Chapter 2], and that's the first time I had ever heard of that. Because of the way my mind was working, something attracted me to it. I wanted something that was that powerful. Remember, I was Superwoman, and I wasn't about to get so crazy. But I wanted what he had.

Soon afterwards, my connection with this guy ended because he found another girl. But by that time I was spending so much money on coke that I needed some way to con people into giving me coke. With men it was easy; if I had sex, I'd get it. I slept with everybody and his brother because I'd always get more coke. I was what they call a coke whore. Everybody knew it, but I didn't care. I was sleeping with guys that I never would have looked at twice. I can't even remember some of the guys that I went to bed with. But as long as they had coke, I thought it was wonderful. At the time, I was really convinced that most of these guys were madly in love with me. I did the drugs and I had the euphoria, so I believed that they really thought I was great.

One guy I slept with was a major dealer named Ray. He had a reputation as the biggest coke fiend around. Of course I was madly in love with him, because he gave me all the coke I wanted and I never had to pay for it. He left town because of legal trouble after a few months, and I met this other guy named Bill. Same story—I came on to him just to get free coke, and he eventually turned me on to freebase. The first time I ever freebased coke, I did one hit and just got a little high, and I left the room disappointed. Later on that night, I did two more hits of freebase and that was it. It took me three hits to be totally into it. It was so much better than snorting lines. It was like a lush, mellow high. After I took a hit of freebase, I'd just lie back on the couch and close my eyes. My heart didn't beat fast, at least not at the beginning. It was great. When I snorted coke, my nose was either runny or stuffy and it would drip down my throat and I'd feel my heart beating. None of that happened when I first freebased.

I freebased for about a year, and after two months I was

physically, emotionally, and psychologically addicted to it. I had a love-hate relationship with cocaine at this point. I loved doing it and I hated coming down. When I started freebasing and there was no more Valium, I literally flipped out when the coke was gone. I couldn't fall asleep, and I would throw things around in my apartment, and I would go up and down on the elevator in the apartment building. I would call people at four or five o'clock in the morning looking for more coke. At that point I started getting into over-the-counter sleeping pills. At four o'clock in the morning, totally freebased out of my brain, I would get in my car, drive to an all-night store, buy a bottle of Sominex, go back to my room, and take all 16 pills in the bottle. Two hours later, I would fall asleep; the pills would finally hit me the next day when I'd wake up incredibly sick.

When the relationship with Bill ended, I was in big money trouble. After a month, I owed one coke dealer $3000 and I had no way to come up with the money. The problem was that dealers knew me, so they would "front" me the coke, meaning that they'd give me the coke with the understanding that I'd pay them later. That only happens when a dealer trusts you, and I had a good rapport with one dealer. I had bought coke from him for four or five months and I always paid, so he eventually started fronting me a gram if I would give him $20 toward it the next day. The thing about coke, though, is that after you get it fronted, it's gone in an hour and you don't want to pay for it the next day. By then, all you want is another gram, and you don't even know how you're going to pay for the first gram that you got fronted. I tried to squeeze a lot of people out of money I owed, and I "borrowed" it from everyone I could, with no intention of paying it back, thinking that I needed the money more than they did. That kind of thinking made all the sense in the world to me at the time.

Eventually, nobody would give me money, and this dealer was threatening me, and I asked this one really sleazy guy for money, and he said that he couldn't lend me the money, but he would have a girlfriend of his give me a call. Anyway, she introduced me to a prostitution ring. I'd sleep with these out-of-town businessmen for $100 and all the coke I wanted. At the time, I thought of myself as a high-class call girl. I had all these wonderful words for it, but the bottom line was that I was a hooker. I really started out because I wanted to pay off my debts, but when I would get to the hotel, these guys would turn me on with coke, and in 15 minutes I would be gone with $100 in my hot little hands. But instead of going back to pay the person that I owed, who was threatening to break my legs, I was so addicted from doing that coke with the businessman that I would go back and buy more from somebody else. While I was doing all of this, for five or six months, I knew what I was doing, but somehow I managed to rationalize to myself that I wasn't doing anything wrong. Even though it was totally against all the morals and values that I had been raised with, I just pretended that I was in a fantasyland, like Alice in Wonderland. I pretended that these were guys that I knew, and that I wanted to go to bed with these guys. I pretended that everything was going to be okay.

I was fired from my job that year. At the end of that year, almost everyone I knew got arrested and I was hiding out from the police with some of the men who paid me to be with them. At this point I weighed 100 pounds. I'm 5'8" tall, so at 100 pounds I was a mess. None of my clothes fit me. I wasn't taking showers. I wasn't going out. I was totally isolating myself in my apartment. I was totally paranoid. People would knock at the door and I would hide under the covers. If the phone rang, I'd jump. I'd hide in the bathroom. I didn't see anybody. My family and friends would say to me that something was wrong, that they were afraid I was having a problem with cocaine. They offered to help, but I'd say, "No, nothing's wrong, I'm fine." I wanted people off my back.

I knew at this point, after I'd been a prostitute, that I had a problem. And I knew the problem was cocaine. I just wanted people off my back. There was a part of me that still wanted to believe that I could do it socially, that I could stop on my own. I'd quit tomorrow. I quit a hundred thousand times. There was a little part of me that wanted to think I could do it, but my gut feeling was, "You're never going to do it, Ellen. You're going to die doing coke." Then you know what I'd think? This is really perverted. I thought that I'd die happy, as if I was happy. I was so miserable. Coke wasn't getting me high at all anymore. I was so paranoid, I used to hear cars drive up and think they were the police. I'd drive on the streets and I'd always be looking out of my windows and mirrors. I always thought the cops were after me. I always thought people were talking about me. I thought people that I owed money to were all getting together to hire a hit man to kill me. I was too paranoid to go into supermarkets. I couldn't go food shopping. I couldn't go into a department store. I always thought people were looking at me. I thought the security people knew I did coke. Everywhere I went I thought people knew by looking at me, that they could tell. I just felt that everybody was after me.

When I did a lot of freebasing, I would think there were bugs crawling on me and I would scratch till I had terrible infections up and down my right arm and leg. That was when I had fingernails. I burned them all off from dipping a cotton ball into rubbing alcohol in order to light a freebase pipe. One night I dipped my nails by accident in rubbing alcohol and they all went up in fire. That flipped me out. Around that time I really thought I should just kill myself. I was in so much trouble with money and so many people were after me and it seemed like I couldn't stop doing coke. I couldn't buy it anymore from anybody. I just started stealing it from a couple of coke dealers I went out with, and when they found out, it was as if everybody was after me.

At this point, I thought, "To hell with it," and I bought three bottles of sleeping pills and took them all. I really wanted this nightmare to end. But before I started to go to sleep, I got scared and got myself to an emergency room. They pumped my stomach and did a blood test that was heavily positive for cocaine. They told me that if I didn't sign into a drug treatment program voluntarily, they'd hospitalize me against my will. Thank God someone took over for me, because I was heading for disaster. That was the last day that I ever used any drug or alcohol. I have been straight for two years now, I'm engaged to be married, I've got a good job, I've got good relationships with my friends and my family, and I can honestly say that I'm a very happy person.

6

Cocaine and the Family

Happy families are all alike; every
unhappy family is unhappy in its own way.
Leo Tolstoy

When 21-year-old Tom A. ran out of money after a cocaine binge, he asked his parents to drive him to New York City to replenish his supply. When they demurred, he threatened to rob a gas station to finance his habit. Mr. and Mrs. A. never found out whether Tom would have carried out his threat, since they gave in to his request. This scenario was repeated on numerous occasions, always with the same result. Tom's parents ultimately sold their home in order to continue supporting their son's habit. As Mrs. A. said, "Whenever I thought of not giving in to him, I imagined him in a shootout with the police and I pictured Tom dead. No matter what, I couldn't let that happen to my boy."

Larry B. was a 32-year-old man who regularly visited prostitutes when using cocaine. His wife had known of his cocaine use and his extramarital affairs for several years, and she had begged him to stop. Shortly after he entered treatment, Larry's wife informed him that she was leaving because of his drug use. Larry responded by saying, "She always says this after she finds out about one of my flings. She'll get over it in a few weeks if I can keep my nose clean. I never worry about her leaving me."

Martha C. was a 36-year-old woman who had used cocaine heavily for three years. Her moods fluctuated rapidly, and she drank heavily in an attempt to "balance out" some of the stimulant effects of cocaine. Her 14-year-old daughter, a former honor-roll student, had recently become truant, had started drinking, had become promiscuous, and had begun experiencing bouts of severe depression.

Cocaine abuse does not occur in a vacuum. For every cocaine abuser, there is a family, which usually suffers greatly. Although the specific behaviors associated with cocaine abuse vary from individual to individual, certain common events wreak havoc on the families of cocaine abusers.

1. Cocaine abusers frequently lie about their whereabouts and their drug use, so that family members can rarely believe anything they say.
2. Cocaine abusers often neglect their usual responsibilities, such as paying bills, remembering appointments, or going to work on time.
3. Cocaine abusers may deplete the family finances. Indeed, the financial problems may become so serious that they will resort to drug dealing, burglary, borrowing from loan sharks, or stealing from the family. It is not an uncommon experience for a cocaine abuser to support his habit by pawning wedding rings, family heirlooms, and other irreplaceable items of high sentimental and often low financial worth. Some individuals resort to stealing their children's savings to support their habits.
4. Cocaine abusers display rapid mood shifts; they may become quite paranoid, believing that individuals around them are plotting against them. The paranoia, which is frequently accompanied by irritability, impulsiveness, and explosiveness, may lead to verbal or physical attacks on family members.
5. Since cocaine is often associated with sexuality, the drug may initially be used in the context of extramarital affairs, thus making the drug use even more distressing to the spouse. In addition, long-term cocaine use frequently causes sexual dysfunction, which can also place great stress on a marriage.

It is easy to see how this pattern of behavioral disturbances can create enormous difficulties within a family. In this chapter, we will discuss the feelings commonly experienced by families of cocaine abusers. We will then discuss some of the ways in which people try to manage life with a cocaine-dependent relative. We will explain how sincere attempts to help the cocaine abuser frequently backfire, and we will recommend ways in which family members can help both themselves and the abuser.

Family Responses to the Cocaine Abuser

Anger

Anger is probably the most common feeling experienced by relatives of cocaine abusers. They feel manipulated, unloved, and abused; they resent playing second fiddle to a drug. Ruth D. summarized the feelings of many spouses of cocaine abusers:

> I used to love my husband. He was a warm, kind, generous man. He loved me and he loved our children. But since he started using cocaine, he has turned into a monster. He screams at me and the children for no reason at all, and he constantly threatens us. He has stolen my jewelry and he went into my daughter's savings account and stole all of her babysitting earnings. The only sex he ever wants is with his coke whores, and because of him, I never answer the phone for fear of being harassed by a bill collector or threatened by a loan shark. I have no love for this man anymore, only hatred.

Guilt

One difficulty that some family members have in experiencing or expressing anger is their profound sense of guilt, which stems from their belief that they are somehow responsible for their relative's continuing drug use. Frequently parents, spouses, and children believe that if they had only acted properly, the addiction would never have occurred. Certainly, most cocaine abusers are happy to accept this theory. They frequently blame their difficulties on their perceived mistreatment by others, rarely accepting the fact that their addiction is responsible for their misfortune. Many family members are only too eager to believe the abuser when he says that his fate is in their hands. By accepting this theory, they believe (mistakenly) that they have some ability to control this terrible illness that is ruining their family.

Fear

As cocaine dependence worsens, family members become increasingly afraid: afraid for their relative, afraid for themselves, and afraid for the family as a whole. As the father of one young cocaine abuser said,

> I never knew from one night to the next what was going to happen. I stayed up till all hours of the night, waiting for her to come home, not sure whether I wanted her to or not. As long as she wasn't home, I knew that something terrible was happening to her, but at least I didn't have to see it. When she did get home, I knew that she wasn't out on the street doing God knows what, but then I would be physically afraid for my wife and myself, because she blamed all of her troubles on us. She went on rampages and threw plates all around the house, and I never knew if she would finally snap and try to kill us.

Shame

As an individual's cocaine dependence worsens, family members frequently become more and more despondent and hopeless. Their feelings about themselves may be characterized by self-blame, inadequacy, and at times self-loathing. They may believe that the cocaine abuser has disgraced the entire family, symbolizing their failure as parents, spouses, or children. One 14-year-old girl whose mother was a cocaine abuser said,

> It got to the point where I couldn't bring other kids over to my house. My mother would sneak around, whispering about people out to get her, and there would always be some strange, sleazy-looking guy hanging around. She was nasty to me and all of my friends, and she used to call me names like "slut" in front of my friends for no reason at all. I'm sure that people must have looked down on me because of my mother, and the only way I knew how

to handle it was to not let friends come over. It's hard to do, though, because after a while, people will stop inviting me over to their houses if I never ask them back. But I don't want to get the reputation as some creep or crazy person because of my mother.

The isolation that this young girl experienced is common in the families of drug abusers and can lead to a great sense of loneliness. As we shall see, this pattern of shame leading to isolation and loneliness is a particularly dangerous one, because it may lead the relative to believe that the only way to rescue his or her own life is by "rescuing" the cocaine abuser. As we shall see, not only is this an impossible task, but—paradoxically—it frequently allows the drug dependence to worsen.

How Families Try to Avoid the Pain of Cocaine Dependence

Denial

When faced with the painful feelings of anger, guilt, fear, and shame, family members frequently seek a way out. The fastest escape from these feelings is the same mechanism used by the abuser: denial. Denial in the family can take many forms. For example, relatives may join in with the abuser's denial by blaming his or her problems on other people, the abuser's job, the police, too much pressure—anything other than cocaine use. One frequent target of this misplaced blame is the family itself. This occurs partly because many relatives accept the role of scapegoat for the addict's difficulties.

Why would a family member accept blame for something that an impartial observer would say he did not cause? Let us give an example that will illustrate this phenomenon and the reasons behind it. Linda D. was a 29-year-old attorney whose cocaine use clearly was causing her difficulties both at work and at home. She was alternately depressed and angry, she frequently missed deadlines at work, she alienated and lost clients, and she fought with her husband about virtually everything. Her husband, a passive and quiet man, rarely made demands on her because he knew it would create strife. He accepted her explanation that excessive job pressure had rendered her unable to cope with even minimal stress. He therefore bent over backwards to lighten her load at home. When he realized that she was using much more cocaine than he had previously believed, he suggested that she cut down. This infuriated her, so he purposely did not bring up the subject again for several months, believing that "nagging" her would only increase her drug use. When he discovered that her cocaine use was escalating anyway, he discussed it with her again and suggested that she seek help. She refused to do so, and began to blame her drug use on her husband's "incessant harping." Although he initially accepted this explanation, he ultimately gained some perspective after she had entered treatment and stopped using cocaine. He described his reaction when she blamed him for her drug problem:

> When she blamed me, it actually gave me a strange sense of hope. I thought, "If this is my fault in some way, then I have the power to make her stop using cocaine." How was that consoling? If I weren't influencing her, then all I could do was watch her throw her life and our marriage away. That prospect was a lot worse than feeling like I had some responsibility for her drug use.

Denial may also occur because relatives do not want to acknowledge that a loved one has a serious drug problem. Since so many people see addiction as an untreatable disease with terrible social stigma attached to it, acknowledgment of such an illness in a family member may initially seem unbearable. Relatives therefore look for an alternative explanation for erratic behavior, difficulties at work, mood swings, paranoia, unexplained weight loss, disappearing money, and odd sleeping habits rather than face the fact that they have an addicted relative. Thus, denial in the family is frequently a defense against fear: fear of helplessness against the disease, and fear of the connotations and consequences of addiction.

Enabling

When the seriousness of an addiction makes denial impossible to maintain, a new pattern of behavior may appear in the family. Because of a strong sense of fear and guilt, relatives may begin to cover up for the patient's addiction, attempting to minimize the consequences that the addicted relative suffers as a result of the drug use. Family members may take over some of the responsibilities of an addicted relative, shield him from creditors, rescue him from drug-related legal difficulties, perhaps going so far as to use drugs with the addict in an attempt to "keep him off the streets." This type of family behavior is generally called *enabling,* because shielding the addict from the adverse consequences of drug use actually supports the addiction.

To understand this last statement, we need to explain why cocaine abusers generally seek treatment. They do not ordinarily stop using the drug merely because they feel they are using "too much." Cocaine is too powerful and too reinforcing to be given up without having compelling reasons for doing so. Therefore, it is frequently necessary for a cocaine abuser to either suffer a meaningful loss or be threatened with such a loss before he will cease his drug use. If a cocaine abuser believes that he can continue to use the drug with impunity, he will be much less likely to stop.

What are some examples of enabling behavior? Dr. Charles Nelson has listed six patterns that are frequently seen in the relatives of cocaine abusers.

1. *Avoiding and Shielding:* This involves an attempt to prevent the abuser from experiencing the adverse consequences of his drug use. Examples include hiding or throwing away cocaine and making up excuses to the abuser's friends and employer in order to cover up his drug use.
2. *Attempting to Control:* This may include a variety of efforts such as screaming, making bargains or threats, leaving the house periodically, withholding sex, buying things for the abuser in order to divert his attention, or constantly staying with him in order to control the amount of his drug use.
3. *Taking Over Responsibilities:* This typically involves taking over a variety of personal responsibilities for the abuser, such as paying bills, performing household tasks, waking the abuser in time for work, or covering debts.
4. *Rationalizing and Accepting:* The relative denies the severity of the drug use; some may even convince themselves that

cocaine has made the abuser more communicative, more sexually attractive, or more creative.

5. *Cooperating and Collaborating:* The relative becomes directly involved with the drug use, helping the user to pay for, prepare, or use cocaine.

6. *Rescuing and Subserving:* This consists of overprotectiveness to the point of making one's own needs secondary to those of the addict. An example of this type of behavior would be cleaning up the cocaine user's vomit after a binge.

Donna T. unsuccessfully tried a variety of enabling behaviors to get her husband Larry to stop his cocaine use. At no time was she aware that her attempts to help him were backfiring. Rather, she felt that the failure of her efforts reflected her inadequacy as a wife. In her words,

I first began to suspect that there was something wrong in our marriage when Larry started going out at night without me. We had always gone out separately once a week with our friends, and I had liked that arrangement. But when he started wanting to go out two or three times a week without me, I suspected that he was seeing another woman. We had only been married three years, but I figured that something had to be missing in our marriage, and I naturally assumed that there was something wrong with me. Why else would a man go out that often without his wife? I never suspected at first that he was using cocaine. I knew that he used it every once in a while, and I had used it socially with him a few times. But it never seemed like a big deal.

I first began to suspect that he had a cocaine problem when we started having money problems. I would ask Larry why there seemed to be so little money left over from his paycheck, and he would just get mad at me and blame me for being a nag. I started getting more and more insecure and tried being nicer to him, figuring that maybe I had been kind of bitchy toward him. I started buying him surprise presents even though we were low on money. I tried to make all of his favorite foods, and I even tried doing different sexual things that I knew he wanted even though I wasn't really comfortable with them. *[At this point, Donna is now subserving herself to her husband. She is also not recognizing her anger at him because of her fear that she is losing him and her guilt that it is her fault.]*

As time went on, it seemed like I couldn't do enough. No matter what I did, he kept going out, and he went out more and more often. When he came home, he would be irritable and would barely talk to me. Meanwhile, I found out that he wasn't paying any bills, although he had always been good about that in the past. We started getting letters from collection agencies and I started getting harassed by bill collectors on the phone. When I brought this up to him, he would just yell at me, so I started paying as many bills as I could out of my own paycheck, hoping that things would somehow straighten out. *[Donna is now taking over responsibilities for her husband, still unaware of what is happening, but clearly afraid for herself and her marriage.]*

One night, Larry didn't come home, and I got really upset. I was sure that he was out with another woman, and I didn't know if I could stand living with him under such circumstances. The next day when he came home, he denied being out with someone else, but admitted that he was using coke. Then he blamed the whole thing on me, saying that I wasn't enough fun, that I was too uptight sexually, and that I wouldn't use cocaine with him, so he had to do it with his friends. I figured that maybe I could help him to control the amount of cocaine he was using if I used some with him. That way, I could keep an eye on him and keep the problem from getting out of hand. *[Donna is now attempting to control his use by cooperating and collaborating with him.]* For a while, I thought things were getting better. Larry seemed a little bit calmer and happier than before, and I figured that at least he wasn't out with other women. *[She is now rationalizing and accepting his use.]*

It didn't take long for things to get really disastrous, though. His habit kept getting bigger and the trouble kept worsening. As he stayed home using his cocaine, we became social recluses. Friends would call us up to do things and I would make up one excuse after another to try to avoid seeing them. *[She is now avoiding and shielding.]* I tried threats, blackmail, bribery, perverted sex, using drugs with him, not using drugs with him, threatening to kill him, threatening to kill myself, leaving the house for a few days—everything I knew in order to get him to stop, but nothing helped. It was as if he didn't even notice that I was alive. Eventually, he started getting into trouble at work, and his boss was a lot more secure than I was. He just told Larry to go into the hospital or give up his job. When it was put that way, Larry checked himself in the next day, because he loved his job and because he knew that his boss meant business.

What is wrong with enabling? There is generally nothing wrong with the motivation behind the behavior or the diligence with which the effort is made. Family members of cocaine addicts are desperate, and they work terribly hard to try to get their relatives to stop using cocaine. However, when they use the methods that Donna used, they are almost always doomed to fail. A term that has been used by some to describe relatives who use these enabling behaviors is *co-dependent*. This term implies that family members are also made ill by the addictive process, and that they themselves need help to recover from the devastating effects of this illness.

Deciding when to "help out" an addicted relative and when to let him fall can be an extremely complicated and painful task for relatives. These issues are illustrated in the following case example. Mr. and Mrs. G. began to suspect that their son, Bob, was in trouble when they noticed money missing from their wallets. They knew that he "fooled around" with drugs, but they did not confront him because they were afraid of what they might find if they delved too deeply. Eventually, Bob was arrested for dealing cocaine; his father hired the best criminal attorney available to defend him. Bob was acquitted, but two months later, he was arrested again on the same charges. He was bailed out of jail by his parents; they hired the same attorney, who was again able to obtain Bob's acquittal. Four days later, Bob was in an intensive care unit, recovering from a cocaine overdose.

Did Mr. and Mrs. G. act wrongly by trying to keep their son out of jail? Would Bob have stopped cocaine sooner if he had not been bailed out of jail and had been forced to accept a public defender? No one can answer this. Bob's parents did what the vast majority of people would have done in the same situation. They tried to keep their son from suffering the possible irreparable harm of incarceration, fervently hoping that he would use his arrests as a warning signal of what might happen to him. They hoped that he would change his behavior in order to avert a worse scenario at a later date.

Unfortunately, events that Mr. and Mrs. G. interpreted as frightening portents were viewed by Bob as evidence of his charmed existence. When asked during treatment about his arrest, he said,

> I knew that nothing was going to happen to me. When I got off after the first bust, it became clear to me that nothing *really* bad was going to happen. Here I was, caught red-handed making a cocaine deal, and I walked away from it. I figured if I could beat that charge, I could beat anything.

The problem with enabling behavior is that it allows the addict to feel omnipotent; it reaffirms what we term the "pathological optimism" of the cocaine abuser: his feeling that he will land on his feet, no matter what happens to him. Since an enabled cocaine abuser does not believe that future use will lead to adverse consequences, he is less likely to stop using the drug.

How Relatives Can Help

Intervention

One of the harmful aspects of enabling behavior is the fact that shielding the cocaine abuser from the adverse consequences of his drug use may allow initially manageable problems to become uncontrollable. Thus, many addicts who have been enabled do not seek treatment until they have suffered irreparable harm: serious physical damage, loss of a valued job, or jail. Meanwhile, their families have been hurt and embittered to an extent that is similarly difficult to repair.

Although some clinicians believe that cocaine abusers do not become motivated to stop their drug use until they "hit bottom" and lose everything, most people in the addictions treatment field believe that this scenario can be avoided through the process of *intervention*. Intervention involves confrontation of the abuser by his family (or employer—see Chapter 7) in order for him to learn how his behavior has adversely affected his own welfare and their lives. At an intervention meeting, family members and friends may gather together with the cocaine abuser and a professional—typically a physician, psychologist, or social worker experienced in such work. They then present the cocaine abuser with: a) clear, nonjudgmental documentation of the results of his substance abuse; b) treatment options that would be acceptable to the family; and c) a clear statement of the family's response if he either refuses treatment or continues his substance abuse.

Interventions are emotionally charged, extremely difficult meetings in which the cocaine abuser often feels attacked and sometimes feels unloved. Family members may worsen the situation by seeing the intervention meeting as their chance to finally obtain revenge on the person who has made their lives so miserable. The presence of a skilled professional is important in such a meeting to ensure that the individual in question really has a substance abuse problem, and to help the addict to hear the genuine concern of his family, not just attacks. When all goes well, the evidence presented may prove overwhelming enough to convince the addict that he has a problem that needs to be taken seriously. Ideally, he may decide to enter treatment immediately. It is therefore important that no intervention take place unless there is an opportunity for immediate placement into treatment, since the impact of the intervention can otherwise be quickly lost.

Another possible outcome of an intervention is that the addict agrees to stop his substance abuse, but refuses to enter any or some of the treatments suggested. Thus, for example, the individual may agree to undergo psychotherapy, but will not attend Narcotics Anonymous or enter a hospital. Alternatively, he may say that he will stop using drugs on his own, without the aid of any sort of treatment. The family should decide prior to the intervention how they will respond if this occurs, since a partial agreement of this nature is a common response. Family members must be ready to state what they will and will not tolerate, and what is and is not negotiable. In some cases, the family may decide to not allow the individual back into the home until he has sought treatment.

A third possible result of an intervention is that the cocaine abuser will continue to deny the seriousness of his drug abuse and will thus refuse to stop using. Although such cases are initially discouraging, many of these families nevertheless benefit from the act of carrying out the intervention. This may represent the first time that family members have attempted honestly and forthrightly to face the reality of their relative's addiction. Since families of addicts are frequently plagued by codes of silence, bickering, scapegoating, and mutual blaming, the opportunity for family members to speak openly about their feelings in a supportive environment can be extremely important. Another helpful aspect of the intervention is the fact that relatives are educated about the effects of substance abuse on the individual and the family. They may also be introduced to sources of ongoing support that are available to them in the community. These include Al-Anon, Nar-Anon, and Coke-

Anon: organizations designed for the family members of individuals with alcohol and drug problems.

Perhaps the most important benefit of the process of intervention is the resolution by family members to stop enabling their relative's addiction. This may involve refusing to pay the addict's bills, refusing to lie in order to protect his social or business reputation, or refusing to live in the same house with him. As one woman said to her husband in an intervention meeting,

> We are offering you one final chance to turn your life around. We have suffered too much as the result of your addiction. We love you and hope that you will get help so that we can live again as a family in peace. If you decide to get treatment, we will support you every step of the way. On the other hand, if you choose to continue using drugs, we have decided that we will no longer support your drug use in any way, because it hurts you and it hurts us. If you decide to return to drugs, then we will focus on getting our own lives together.

Taking such a stand can initiate recovery for the family, and may eventually help the cocaine abuser to seek help himself.

Recovery for the Families of Cocaine Abusers

Although it may be quite dramatic, an intervention represents only the beginning of the long-term recovery process for the cocaine abuser and his family. Cessation of cocaine use does not remove the memories, distrust, and pain that occurred during periods of active drug abuse. Recovery also creates the need for adjustments in the family, because relatives have learned to adapt to life with an addict. For example, family members who endure chronic chaos and abuse may develop a sense of pride in their ability to tolerate disaster. They may thus feel less "special" when their burden is taken away from them. Relatives may also become quite resentful when the addict starts to regain some self-esteem and begins to feel good about himself soon after entering treatment. As the spouse of one cocaine abuser said, "How dare he feel so proud of himself after he has ruined my life for the last five years?" Some who have been hurt by their addicted relatives want revenge, but they rarely find satisfaction in the process.

For these and other reasons, support for family members of

cocaine abusers is extremely important, both for them and for the recovery of the addict. This may consist of psychotherapy, counseling, or Al-Anon, Nar-Anon, or Coke-Anon meetings. The latter groups support relatives of substance abusers by encouraging them to take care of themselves rather than trying to take care of their addicted relatives. These meetings, which can be attended by relatives or friends of active or recovering substance abusers, are guided by the same 12-step recovery program as Alcoholics Anonymous and Narcotics Anonymous. One of the most important guiding principles is the first step to recovery: "We admitted we were powerless over alcohol [drugs, cocaine]—that our lives had become unmanageable." Members of Al-Anon are encouraged to resist enabling by reminding themselves of the "three C's": they did not *cause* their relative's addiction, nor can they *control* or *cure* it. They are thus encouraged to "detach with love": to gain control over their own lives by realizing their inability to control the life of the addict.

Lasting recovery does not come easily. Family members must be prepared to deal with relapses on the part of the abuser and their own temptation to return to familiar but maladaptive coping mechanisms such as enabling. Relatives may try to "protect" the recovering addict from stress because of their fear that he will return to drugs if they become upset with him. Families who have argued constantly for years may not know how to interact when there is nothing to fight about. Some of these problems can be dealt with in ongoing family meetings, led by a professional who is experienced in family therapy. Families who have never communicated honestly and openly frequently need help and support in order to begin and continue this process. The following case example illustrates one of the common pitfalls in the recovery process for families. In cases such as this, family therapy can help heal the wounds caused by chronic drug abuse.

Barbara E., a 26-year-old woman with a history of cocaine addiction, had been drug-free for one year. She was successful in her career and lived in her own apartment. She and her parents attended family therapy together because of the great difficulty they had experienced in talking to each other after her parents had learned of her cocaine use. At one meeting, Mrs. E. said, "I'm scared to put pressure on Barbara because I'm afraid she won't be able to handle it." This occurred shortly after Barbara had told her mother about a very painful problem she had endured with her boyfriend, an incident that she had handled with great aplomb and maturity. Barbara became quite upset and said, "Mom, you're doing now what you accused me of doing for years, which was not speaking my true feelings. You don't talk to me about painful stuff because *you* can't handle it." Mrs. E. was encouraged to speak more honestly and openly to her daughter, and to worry less about Barbara's fragility. With time, she was able to do so, and was pleased to see that both she and Barbara could tolerate such an exchange.

7

Cocaine in the Workplace

Until recently, the high cost of cocaine served to limit its use to people who either had substantial disposable income or were selling the drug. As a result, publicity about cocaine abusers has tended to focus on entertainers and professional athletes who have come to public attention in a variety of ways: some after being arrested for cocaine-related crimes (e.g., dealing or possession), others after their careers or personal lives have been shattered or ended by cocaine use.

The recently decreased price and increased availability of cocaine has done a great deal to alter this picture. People without great wealth are now finding cocaine affordable. Thus, cocaine has found its way into many areas of society, including the workplace. Indeed, surveys reveal that with the exception of alcohol, cocaine is fast becoming the most prevalent drug of abuse among those who use drugs in a work setting. The growing number of referrals of cocaine abusers to employee assistance programs and drug treatment programs tends to confirm this impression. Indeed, according to some studies, the cost of cocaine use in lost productivity, job-related accidents, claims for health care benefits, and poor employee morale may be over 10 billion dollars a year.

As cocaine use spreads beyond professional athletes and entertainers to individuals in all walks of society, it is inevitable that the drug will be (and has been) used by occupational groups in whom cocaine intoxication presents a danger not only to the user but to the general public as well. Specifically, occupations with long hours and high levels of tension, intermixed with boredom, provide fertile ground for the development of on-the-job cocaine use. As a result, air traffic controllers, pilots, workers in nuclear power plants, ambulance drivers, physicians, and nurses have all been noted to be at high risk for cocaine abuse.

Why Cocaine?

The reasons for cocaine's intrusion into the workplace relate both to social factors and to the properties of the drug itself. Certainly, the frequent revelation that celebrities in our society are also cocaine users has helped to endow the drug with a certain mystique. Its use by potential role models has also helped sanctify and glamorize its use for certain members of society. The latter include a variety of social climbers, "groupies," and status-conscious young adults who grew up in the drug culture of the 1960s and 1970s, whose earlier experiences with marijuana, hallucinogens, and alcohol have prepared them for subsequent experimentation with other drugs. Indeed, within some peer groups, cocaine use has become a socially sanctioned—and at times expected—social behavior, much the way alcohol use is for other segments of our society.

Cocaine use in the workplace is facilitated by the fact that quantities sufficient to produce multiple episodes of intoxication can be transported in a small vial or aspirin bottle. In addition, the act of consuming the drug can be accomplished in seconds, with intoxication occurring almost instantaneously. Moreover, individuals who are "high" on cocaine frequently believe that despite being intoxicated, they are capable of "normal" functioning, both interpersonally and intellectually. Most importantly, they believe that their intoxication is not apparent to those around them. In contrast, use of drugs like heroin, hallucinogens, or phencyclidine (PCP) is commonly known to render the user nonfunctional and thus easily detectable.

Another appealing property of cocaine is the fact that its use in low to moderate doses generally produces euphoria, increased alertness, and a sense of well-being. As a result, difficult tasks may seem easier, and boring repetitive tasks can be performed more rapidly. Jobs that require sustained attention can also be done more quickly, although far less carefully.

Hazards of Cocaine Use in the Workplace

Cocaine use, in either a social or occupational setting, is not without hazards, many of which have been described in previous chapters. In this chapter, we will focus on the drug's effect on work performance and relationships with co-workers. The following case illustrates some points about how the development of cocaine dependence can be both facilitated and interrupted by work-related factors.

> Carl, a 30-year-old car salesman, entered treatment because of a three-year history of cocaine abuse. He had reluctantly agreed to seek help at the insistence of his father, who owned the car dealership in which he worked. His father accompanied him to the initial appointment. Although Carl initially stated that he used cocaine only for "recreational" purposes on weekends, he grudgingly admitted that within the last three months, he had begun using the drug at work and that this had perhaps interfered with his performance. His father was more definite, characterizing the last several months as a financial and social disaster.
>
> The youngest of three siblings, Carl described himself as a shy young man who had had aspirations to be a teacher. He was discouraged from pursuing a teaching career by his father and two older brothers, all of whom worked successfully in the family's automobile dealership. His inability to assert himself within the family was paralleled by awkwardness in social situations, particularly with women. Three years ago, he was offered cocaine at a party and reluctantly agreed to try the drug so that others would not feel that he was a "wimp." He enjoyed the euphoria and sense of increased confidence he experienced after taking the drug. Subsequently, he used cocaine again in similar circumstances on weekends.
>
> As time passed, Carl's cocaine use increased in frequency from once or twice a month to every weekend. It was particularly heavy prior to, and during, social occasions. He felt the drug made him more assertive and, as a result, he was more comfortable with women. He also noted that while on cocaine, he was able to be more assertive with his father and brothers and felt less "pushed around" by them. These experiences reinforced his be-

lief that for him, cocaine had a useful therapeutic effect.

As Carl's weekend cocaine use increased, he noted that Mondays were difficult, in that he experienced low mood, fatigue, and difficulty concentrating on his work. Although he did not associate these difficulties with cocaine withdrawal, he began using a "line" or two on Monday mornings to "get going." He then noted that he was becoming more assertive and selling more cars. He was soon named "salesman of the month," thereby winning the respect of his father and brothers.

Over the next six months, Carl's cocaine use gradually increased in frequency to the point where he was using the drug several times a day. His fellow workers began to note that in addition to being more assertive, he was also somewhat irritable and suspicious. His abrasiveness began to offend potential customers, some of whom complained to his father. His drug use on weekends also increased so that from Friday night to Monday morning, he was almost continuously intoxicated. Moreover, whereas cocaine had previously enhanced his ability to socialize, he now preferred to use the drug while alone in his room, emerging only to replenish his supply or to meet with other friends who were also cocaine users. A newly found girlfriend left him, telling his brothers that he was "acting weird" and that on several occasions he had been physically violent toward her as a result of cocaine-induced paranoia. At this point, his family confronted him about his drug use, which he minimized. Finally, at a stormy business meeting, he was confronted about his dwindling sales and poor attitude. He reluctantly agreed to seek help as an alternative to being fired.

This case illustrates some typical features in the development of cocaine abuse. Many individuals who experience uncertainty in interpersonal situations, who have difficulty "standing up" to their boss, or who feel chronically "put down" find that cocaine elevates mood, raises their self-esteem, and provides a false sense of security in interpersonal situations. Thus, in the beginning, cocaine use may actually help in overcoming real or imagined problems with initiative, assertiveness, or self-confidence. As a result, there is a tendency to turn to cocaine repeatedly in times of stress and to impart to the drug healing or restorative powers. Over time, however, the number of work-related or social situations that "require" pretreatment with cocaine increases to the point where the user feels totally unable to function properly without being intoxicated.

As the cocaine user is gradually seduced, he may begin to lose sight of the drug's detrimental effects on work performance. The personality changes that accompany cocaine use (see Chapters 4 and 5) and the financial burden imposed by regular use also take their toll. In particular, there is the tendency of long-term users to develop significant dependence on the drug. Such individuals, even if not intoxicated at work, may spend their work day preoccupied with obtaining cocaine or anticipating its use. As in the case of Carl, they may also begin to experience the rebound depression that often accompanies cocaine withdrawal. This in turn causes them to use the drug in the morning before going to work.

As anticipated or actual drug use occupies more and more of the work day, there is a corresponding fall-off in work performance as users experience drug effects, drug withdrawal, or apprehension about being caught. Despite these complications, users typically feel that they are functioning as well as, if not better than, they did prior to the onset of regular use. However, their supervisors frequently do not share this view. Thus, it comes as a great surprise when they are passed over for promotion or fired outright as a result of sloppy work performance or deteriorating personal relationships with fellow employees and clients.

This case also illustrates the potential power of an *intervention* (see Chapter 6) in the workplace, in which an employee is confronted about his drug use by his supervisor(s) and is required to either enter treatment or lose his job. Carl, like many other cocaine abusers, was able to admit to his problem only after being confronted in this manner.

Cocaine Use by Executives

Although drug abuse per se has traditionally been regarded as a problem for people in the lower socioeconomic classes, there is growing recognition that the problem is not confined to any social group. Indeed, data from employee assistance programs and drug rehabilitation centers are showing that drug abuse by executives and professionals is on the rise. Moreover, users include not only young middle managers but corporate directors as well. Although alcohol is still the most common drug of abuse in this population, cocaine abuse is increasing dramatically in this segment of the work force.

Why would an otherwise successful business executive be attracted by the lure of cocaine? The popularity of cocaine among business executives stems from a variety of factors. These include the easy transportability of the drug, the fact that it can be self-administered within a matter of seconds in a locked office or bathroom, and the widespread misconception that cocaine intoxication does not interfere with intellectual functioning or decision making. In addition, for some executives, cocaine's ability to elevate mood and enhance their feelings of competence makes the drug appear to be a useful adjunct in their attempts to impress a co-worker or a board of directors. Moreover, the hyperactivity and grandiosity that often accompany long-term cocaine use do little to contradict this self-perception. Unfortunately, supervisors, fellow employees, and competitors frequently see things otherwise.

Another factor that may contribute to cocaine use by executives is that a growing number of them are members of the "baby boom" generation of the post-World War II era. This population group, which is now entering its middle years, has had substantial experience with the use of other psychoactive drugs. In the 1960s, when they were adolescents and young adults, recreational use of marijuana and hallucinogens may have been socially acceptable within their peer group. For many, getting a job, marrying, and having children have not altered this view. This is particularly true in the large urban areas of both coasts, where young and middle-aged professionals congregate around universities and high-technology industry. Here there exists a social milieu that is basically a continuation of their college experience, where willingness to experiment with new "recreational" drugs, like cocaine, is socially acceptable. In contrast to opiates or sedatives, which render the user nonfunctional for at least an hour or two, cocaine is seen as a drug that enhances social relationships.

In many respects, the upwardly mobile young executive is an inviting target for cocaine use. Job pressures, long hours, frequent travel, and fierce competition each take their toll, not only on the individual but on his or her major sources of emotional support: family and friends. In the business world, being a good spouse or parent are virtues that often go unrecognized and unrewarded. Although lip service is paid to the value of recreation, "quality time" with family members, and the need for rewarding nonbusiness relationships, the intense competitiveness of the business world often makes such activities seem frivolous. Sometimes, cocaine use is initiated as a substitute for meaningful family or marital relationships. Not surprisingly, some successful executives experience themselves as increasingly isolated, with job-related achievement being their only measure of self-worth. In this context, the availability of a drug that promises not only to enhance work performance, but also to make emotional support unnecessary, is a powerful attraction.

With the transition from recreational to habitual cocaine use, the focus of one's energies gradually turns away from concerns about work or family life and toward ensuring one's cocaine supply. In the workplace, there is a tendency toward increased sharing of information with other users about sources of supply. Joint purchases are made with co-workers in order to avoid low-level street dealers and the risk of being "ripped off," arrested, or blackmailed. As preoccupation with cocaine accelerates, work performance begins to suffer, although the cocaine abuser may be unaware that his judgment and abilities are not what they should be. When criticized by others, the abuser may be defensive, perhaps paranoid. Some individuals begin to feel that supervisors or co-workers are conspiring against them; sometimes they are right.

A business executive in trouble with cocaine frequently finds himself with no one to turn to. After several years of drug involvement have complicated what may have already been a difficult marital relationship, the cocaine abuser's spouse may no longer be emotionally available. In other instances, the spouse may also be a drug or alcohol abuser, and may thus be unable to offer emotional support when needed. The executive may then attempt to use cocaine as a "bargaining chip" in exchange for friendship, emotional support, or sexual favors from co-workers. A common scenario is the middle-aged businessman who begins to supply cocaine to his secretary or someone else lower on the corporate ladder. This may be a way of enlisting allies in a real or imagined corporate struggle or an attempt to recapture lost youth in a relationship based on drugs and sex. Some business subordinates may find cocaine use intoxicating and exciting, while others are intimidated enough to go along with it despite their better judgment.

The Response of Business

In addition to the personal costs of cocaine use, business losses due to drug-related decreases in productivity and faulty decision making probably run in the billions of dollars annually. In addition to its high personal cost, cocaine dependence imposes a heavy financial burden. As a result, users with access to company funds may divert these for their own use through embezzlement, double billing, or acceptance of bribes or kickbacks. In addition, managers whose decisions can influence stock prices or the cost of a company's goods or services may become targets for personal or corporate blackmail when their drug-related impairment becomes known to drug dealers or business competitors. Thus, for the company that employs them, drug-abusing employees are a liability.

The high cost attached to drug abuse in the workplace has prompted the business community to respond in a variety of ways. Some organizations have adopted the posture that drug-abusing employees should be quickly identified and fired. Accordingly, their efforts have focused on detection of users, followed by removal of these employees from the company by whatever means necessary. The detection armamentarium has included random urine screening for drugs of abuse, periodic examination of workers for telltale signs of drug abuse (e.g., needle tracks), paid company informants distributed throughout the work force, and, in some instances, private detectives who spy on workers during and after hours. Such a policy toward drug users, however, has its direct and indirect costs. Employees in such businesses, whether they are drug users or not, frequently feel that the company is dealing with them in an adversarial fashion. This in turn lowers morale and drives the drug problem and other difficulties underground. Employees who might otherwise seek help tend to focus on company harassment rather than on their own problems. Fearing discovery, those who do seek help may do so at their own expense rather than using company-financed insurance benefits. However, since their ability to pay for drug abuse treatment on their own may be limited, they may be more likely to drop out of treatment prematurely.

Another problem with the "detection" approach is that the ubiquitous nature of drug abuse in the workplace makes the monitoring of employees practical only for smaller companies. Organizations with a large work force and multiple work sites have generally found attempts at "weeding out" drug-abusing employees both impractical and costly. Moreover, in replacing such employees, there is little to guarantee that yet another drug abuser will not be hired as a replacement.

In some work settings, the use of illicit drugs, including cocaine, represents a risk not only to the employee and his company, but to the general public as well. Examples include bus and taxi drivers, airline pilots, nurses, physicians, police, and other professions in which public safety is jeopardized by the presence of an intoxicated worker. In such cases, preemployment urine testing for drugs of abuse is sometimes used. Moreover, if there is reason to suspect ongoing drug abuse, random urine screening may serve as both a deterrent and a method of detection. Indeed, some companies are beginning to require urine testing after a work-related accident, absences for undocumented illness, or following a perceived decrement in work performance. In the absence of more subjective measures, however, reliance solely on the results of urine testing can be both clinically and legally hazardous. For example, individuals who have used marijuana consistently can produce urine specimens with detectable levels of tetrahydrocannabinol (THC), marijuana's active ingredient, for over a month after stopping the drug. Indeed, positive tests for THC have been reported in individuals who have merely been in a room where marijuana was smoked. Another difficulty with urine screening programs is deciding how to deal with the presence of drugs that are part of a medically prescribed treatment regimen (e.g., codeine-containing cough preparations), but that may also be abused. Finally, it should be noted that urine and blood tests are not foolproof; both false-positive and false-negative results can occur. Thus, all positive tests should be rechecked with a confirmatory test using a different analytic

method, such as gas chromatography–mass spectrometry
(GC–MS). Tests that remain positive require medical follow-up
to determine whether further action, such as referral for treatment, is necessary.

The use of urine screening to detect drug-using employees is
also complicated by civil rights issues. Not uncommonly, employees have refused to participate in blood or urine testing
programs out of a sense of embarrassment or mistrust. Many
are concerned about issues of confidentiality in the event of a
positive test, and some have brought lawsuits against companies when the companies have taken punitive action on the
basis of tests that the employees claimed were merely false-
positive.

The need for a practical approach to the problem of substance abuse in the workplace does not negate the need for
firm limits on drug-using behavior. Many substance abusers,
like Carl (see pages 109–110), fail to appreciate the severity of
their problem, and some fail to realize that a problem exists. As
a result, they may need to be directly confronted not only by
friends and family members but by their employers as well. In
this context, having to choose between getting help for a drug
problem or losing one's job often provides the needed motivation to seek treatment. Under these circumstances, some companies require objective evidence that the employee is en-
rolled in a treatment program, while others require ongoing
random urine screening for drugs of abuse. In such cases,
urine samples may either be obtained through an outside treatment program or through the employee health clinic as a condition of continuing employment. Usually the company re-
serves the right to suspend or terminate any employee whose
urinalysis indicates the continuation of illicit drug use. In some
instances, the cycle of drug abuse needs to be interrupted by a
brief period of hospitalization, a subject that we will discuss
further in Chapter 8.

The Concept of Employee Assistance

In the absence of a clear company policy that views substance
abuse and other mental health problems as medical/psychi-
atric disorders (rather than moral infirmities), there is a ten-

dency for supervisors either to look the other way when they suspect drug use or to harass suspected employees until they quit or transfer and become someone else's problem. In such an atmosphere, reporting may be precluded by a shortage of skilled workers, favoritism, or fear that one's own drug use will be exposed. Alternatively, peers may cover up for a drug-abusing co-worker so that the supervisor may be unaware of the problem. Eventually, however, absenteeism, poor work performance, and on-the-job intoxication present an overwhelming burden for co-workers and an unacceptable risk for the company.

In some organizations, the emphasis has recently shifted from dismissal of troubled employees to attempts at primary and secondary prevention of illness. Primary prevention efforts include wellness and stress management programs and other attempts to improve the general level of health and well-being of employees. Secondary prevention efforts are focused on the early identification and treatment of troubled employees. Some may already be involved in drug or alcohol abuse; others may be at increased risk for substance abuse as a result of associated mental health problems (such as depression) or a high level of life stress (such as recent separation or divorce).

In an attempt to provide early identification and treatment for troubled employees with substance abuse or other mental health problems, a number of companies have developed, or contracted with, employee assistance programs (EAPs). These companies have decided that the cost of providing treatment for substance abuse or mental impairment in their employees is far less than the decreased productivity caused by these problems. The types of employee assistance available include telephone hotlines run by either paid counselors or volunteers, clinics that offer information and evaluation services to troubled employees and refer them for treatment outside the company, and in-house programs that provide comprehensive medical and psychological services. Today, over 5000 companies, including many Fortune 500 businesses, have functioning EAPs.

Despite the prevalence of EAPs, there have heretofore been few attempts to measure their effectiveness. Many barriers stand between the EAP and its use by employees. Many compa-

nies, including some with EAPs, view mental health problems—and particularly drug and alcohol problems—as a
moral rather than a medical issue. Not surprisingly, some employees feel that if they seek help for emotional or drug-related
problems, their confidentiality will be violated, their promo-
tions will be jeopardized, and they may be fired. Although
many EAPs rely on drug treatment programs that are independent of the company, confidentiality nevertheless remains an
issue. Finally, in some instances, there is a lack of "marketing"
of EAP services, so that employees are only dimly aware of the
kinds of help available.

Despite their inherent difficulties, EAPs appear to be generally helpful. By making evaluation and treatment services
available to drug-dependent employees, EAPs also help to decrease the spread of substance abuse throughout their companies. Since drug-abusing employees are also frequently suppli-
ers of illicit drugs, they are essentially "carriers" of the disease.
The presence of rampant drug use within a company not only
attracts other drug users as job applicants, but also sets up an
atmosphere in which criminal activity may flourish. Prevention, early detection, and treatment efforts help to avert such
situations.

When they work well, EAPs provide a valuable resource for
drug-abusing employees and their supervisors. Ideally, they
provide confidential evaluation and either on-site treatment or
appropriate referral. They provide support and encouragement for employees undergoing active rehabilitation, and they
serve as a link between the treatment program and the workplace. Thus, the efficacy of treatment can be correlated with
work performance. EAPs may, in addition, arrange for in-
house meetings of Alcoholics Anonymous or Narcotics Anonymous for employees in varying stages of recovery from drug
and alcohol dependence. EAP personnel may also establish
close relationships with treatment programs in the community, thus allowing them not only to evaluate the results of
treatment, but to identify the most appropriate treatment re-
sources for their company's employees. Some EAPs also provide evaluation and referral for problems arising within the
employee's family. These may include financial difficulties,
marital infidelity, child abuse, and a host of other drug-related

problems. Individual, couple, and family therapy may be indicated along with the use of outpatient support groups like Alcoholics Anonymous, Narcotics Anonymous, Al-Anon, Nar-Anon, and Alateen.

The EAP also provides a mechanism for monitoring both treatment compliance and post-treatment work performance. As a result, drug-abusing employees are less likely to "fall between the cracks." The existence of a monitoring component within the company also prevents supervisors from transferring problem employees to other parts of the company without revealing the nature of their problem. The latter is common practice in dealing with a disgruntled employee who denies drug use and who threatens to sue the company when he fails to get a desired promotion or when his employment is terminated. In short, a well-functioning EAP can provide a constructive alternative for addressing the problem of drug abuse in the workplace. This, in turn, fosters an atmosphere of concern and caring, rather than an adversarial relationship between the employee and the company.

In summary, the use of illicit drugs—particularly cocaine—is a growing problem, both for drug users and the companies that employ them. The response of management to this problem will do much to determine whether the work environment is one that fosters the initiation and maintenance of drug use or whether it is "therapeutic," in that it provides the structure and level of satisfaction necessary to facilitate the rehabilitation process. What is clear at present is that business cannot afford to ignore the problem of drug abuse in the workplace, and management needs to develop policies and procedures to address it. Approaches that consider the rights and best interests of employees, as well as those of the company, hold the most promise for success. Punitive approaches, which rely solely on detection and termination of employees, merely drive the problem underground; in the long run, such programs are not likely to be cost-effective. The ubiquitous nature of substance abuse in our society makes consideration of these issues of paramount importance for the business community. Hopefully, they will respond to the challenge with creative solutions.

8

Treatment of Cocaine Abuse

Because the current cocaine epidemic is a recent phenomenon, relatively little has been written about the specific treatment of cocaine abuse. Moreover, studies that evaluate various treatments by following up patients after treatment ends have generally been short-term. Unlike studies of alcoholism and heroin addiction that have been carried out over several years, most cocaine treatment studies have covered only six-month periods. Currently, most treatment for cocaine abuse takes place in general drug and alcohol treatment programs, which utilize the same techniques in treating cocaine abusers as in the treatment of patients who are dependent upon other substances. Therefore, although we will review some specific studies of cocaine abuse treatment later in this chapter, most of what we will be describing as treatment for cocaine abuse is based on guiding principles that have been established for the treatment of a wide variety of addictive disorders.

One inherent difficulty in discussing the treatment of cocaine abuse is the fact that most people who use cocaine never seek treatment. Some people try the drug once or twice to satisfy their curiosity, and then never use it again. Others take the drug infrequently, perhaps on special occasions, and suffer no apparent adverse consequences. Still others experience temporary difficulties because of cocaine and decide to stop using the drug on their own. Thus, a significant number of individuals stop using cocaine either because it does too little for them or because they are afraid that it may do too much to them. We could learn a great deal about stopping cocaine use from those who quit the drug on their own: what motivated them, how they did it, what helped. Unfortunately, however, since these individuals do not seek treatment, they have not been formally studied. Such research would be extremely valuable, since the individuals seen in drug abuse treatment centers may represent only a fraction of the overall cocaine picture.

What is the best treatment approach for those who cannot quit by themselves? Unfortunately, we cannot offer a single treatment prescription for all cocaine abusers. People who develop problems with cocaine are individuals, and they need treatment programs that are tailored to fit their own specific needs. While certain people are able to stop using cocaine on their own, some require inpatient hospitalization. Others can be successfully treated as outpatients. In this chapter, we will 1) discuss how and why cocaine abusers enter treatment, 2) describe the various types of treatment methods that are available, and 3) review some of the general principles involved in helping people to stop using cocaine.

Getting the Cocaine Abuser into Treatment

The first requirement of a successful cocaine abuse treatment program is that the patient enters treatment. Unfortunately, this may also be the most difficult aspect of treatment. As we discussed in Chapter 5, cocaine addicts frequently deny or minimize the extent to which their drug use is adversely affecting their lives. Thus, they may not seek treatment until some event begins to break down that denial. Cocaine abusers do not ordinarily seek help merely because they feel they are using too much cocaine. Rather, they usually come to professional attention only after their cocaine abuse is undeniably creating a problem in some other aspect of their lives. Typically, cocaine use causes problems in one of the following areas, any of which may lead the user to seek treatment.

1. *Medical:* Since cocaine abusers are able to deny the importance of such "minor" difficulties as a perforated nasal septum, it may take a major, life-threatening medical problem,
   such as a grand mal seizure (convulsion), to alert the addict
   to the seriousness of the problem.
2. *Vocational:* Absenteeism, tardiness, and erratic job performance are common consequences of cocaine abuse. As
   employers learn more about substance abuse, they are
   more likely to recognize these patterns of behavior as potential symptoms of cocaine abuse. They may respond by making continued employment contingent upon successful
   completion of a drug treatment program.
3. *Financial:* Cocaine is expensive. Unless one is extremely
   wealthy or willing to undertake illegal activity, it is very
   difficult to maintain even a moderate cocaine habit. Unfortunately, some people do not enter treatment until they
   have fallen heavily into debt. For those who fund their habits with criminal activity, legal problems may lead them to
   seek treatment.
4. *Legal:* If you are not rich, the three major methods of main-
   taining a substantial cocaine habit are stealing, dealing, and
   prostitution. Thus, many people enter treatment via the
   criminal justice system. One might instinctively think that
   such individuals would be unmotivated for treatment and
   have a relatively poor prognosis. However, this is not always
   the case, as we will discuss later.
5. *Interpersonal:* As we discussed in Chapter 6, cocaine abuse
   can cause great damage to the family. Sometimes, the only
   leverage that a spouse can exercise in dealing with an addicted partner is the threat of separation. Sometimes, such a
   threat will lead a cocaine abuser into treatment. More often,
   however, the addict finds the threat unbelievable. If the
   ultimatum is being made for the first time, the addict is
   likely to call the spouse's bluff. When threats have been
   made previously but not carried out, then the addict has
   "proof" in his own mind that he has no need to worry.
6. *Psychological:* Some people seek treatment because they
   are frightened of what cocaine is doing to them. They are
   worried by the direct drug effects (depression, hallucinations, paranoia, delusions), and they are frightened by the

erosion of their own values. For example, one patient came to our unit recently because he had overextended himself financially, and he was becoming increasingly tempted to sell his mother's jewelry to finance his habit. Fortunately, his level of denial and rationalization was not high enough to allow him to carry this out, and he sought treatment before he actually completed this act.

Sometimes friends, family members, employers, physicians, or others who are close to a cocaine addict do not wait for him to "hit bottom." Rather, they perform an *intervention*, the purpose of which is to help the addict to face the consequences of his own use. (Interventions are described in more detail in Chapters 6 and 7.) If this is unsuccessful, it may be helpful to create some adverse consequences in a controlled setting before the abuser loses so much that recovery becomes even more difficult. This process is sometimes referred to as "raising the bottom."

Unfortunately, just because an addict comes into treatment does not mean that he is a willing participant. Many of the aforementioned avenues into treatment are at least partially coercive; a major goal of treatment, therefore, is to instill some motivation into the patient. Even in our inpatient setting, in which we require the patient to call the hospital himself in order to formally request admission, the majority of the patients coming into our unit would initially like nothing better than to get high. This is more easily understood when one realizes that most active cocaine addicts want to stop and most abstinent addicts want to get high. What separates the two groups is the relative strengths of these conflicting emotions and, more importantly, the behavioral result of this inner battle. Thus, many of our successful patients leave the hospital after approximately four weeks with the *desire* to get high, but with the ability to not act on this wish.

Treatment Methods for Cocaine Abusers

Outpatient Treatment

The first major question one must answer in considering various treatment methods for a cocaine abuser is whether the drug problem can be managed on an outpatient basis or whether the abuser will need to be hospitalized. Obviously, outpatient treatment is preferable to hospitalization whenever feasible, since it requires the expenditure of considerably less time and money, and minimizes overall life disruption. On the other hand, inpatient treatment has the advantage of being far more intensive, and it removes the addict from what is often a harmful life-style and from ready access to additional cocaine. In assessing an individual's capacity to successfully enter outpatient treatment, we carefully examine the patient's level of denial and his commitment to treatment. In our experience, outpatient treatment has the best chance of success for patients who clearly recognize the destructive impact of cocaine on their lives, and who enter treatment with a sincere desire to do whatever is necessary to stop using the drug. We may initially attempt outpatient treatment with such patients, with the understanding that continued drug use may indicate the need for hospitalization. We ordinarily recommend hospitalization initially for people with questionable motivation and for those whose cocaine use is accompanied by extremely dangerous or self-destructive behavior.

Within the broad category of "outpatient treatment" are numerous specific treatment methods that have been used with varying degrees of success on cocaine abusers and other drug-dependent individuals. In the following section, we will discuss some of the most widely utilized techniques for treating cocaine abusers.

Individual Psychotherapy. In individual psychotherapy, a patient and a psychotherapist (usually a psychiatrist, psychologist, or social worker) discuss a wide variety of personal problems, including the patient's drug use, difficulties with interpersonal relationships, and inner conflicts. Psychotherapy may focus on current life issues or may examine in depth the contribution of childhood experiences to current psychological difficulties. In general, psychotherapy with an active or newly abstinent cocaine abuser is likely to focus primarily on his current difficulties, at least at first. When stable abstinence has brought these crises under control, then further exploration of the origins of the patient's problems can proceed more smoothly.

Paul A., a 31-year-old accountant, entered psychotherapy after his wife told him to either seek treatment for his cocaine abuse or leave the house. He had been treating his wife and son cruelly, was neglecting responsibilities at work, and had experienced numerous bouts of depression. The major focus of his first two months of psychotherapy was stopping his cocaine use. His therapist encouraged Paul to attend Narcotics Anonymous meetings, and they discussed the feelings, events, and places that stimulated his desire for cocaine. Paul's therapist also taught him techniques that could help him avoid drug use even when his craving for cocaine was high.

As Paul's preoccupation with cocaine diminished with a lengthening period of abstinence, the focus of his psychotherapy began to shift toward the initial precipitants for his drug use: anxiety about becoming a father (he began heavy cocaine use during his wife's pregnancy), and his own unresolved relationship with his abusive alcoholic father. As he began to learn more about these issues, he gained a greater sense of mastery over his emotions, and his desire to escape from uncomfortable feelings decreased.

Group Psychotherapy. In group psychotherapy, six to 12 group members meet with one or two professional leaders to discuss both individual problems and relationships among themselves. Groups for drug-dependent patients usually offer peer support for remaining abstinent, advice on such issues as marital and vocational problems, and confrontation when group members perceive that someone is at risk to relapse. One advantage of the group approach is the fact that drug-dependent patients are adept at recognizing subtle signs of denial and self-deceit in each other, since they are so familiar with these behaviors themselves. One potential drawback of group therapy is the fact that some very passive patients who find it difficult to talk in groups may not deal adequately with their own personal problems in this setting.

Steve L., a 22-year-old student, was referred for drug-oriented group psychotherapy because of a history of cocaine abuse and manipulative behavior. Since he was one of the youngest members of the group, he initially tried to impress other group members by recounting "war stories" of his drug use; he reveled in describing his narrow escapes from arrest and serious injury. Other members of the group recognized his high level of anxiety and denial; they therefore offered him a useful combination of support and confrontation. As the group progressed, Steve attempted to exploit other group members, as he had done previously in other relationships. When the group members reacted negatively to this, he began to appreciate the adverse consequences of his manipulativeness. He subsequently made an effort to deal with others more honestly and genuinely.

Couple or Family Therapy. This treatment modality is particularly helpful in families for whom drug use has replaced or precluded other forms of communication. In some families, anger and resentment over one person's substance abuse can severely compromise the ability of family members to talk to one another about anything. In family or couple therapy, various members of a family congregate with a professional family therapist who helps to improve communication patterns within the family, to examine how family stresses are sometimes expressed by one person's drug use, and to help ease the difficulties that the drug abuser and the family both experience during recovery. (Further discussion of family therapy can be found in Chapter 6.)

Medication. The use of medications in the treatment of cocaine abuse has recently been the subject of intense interest. As scientists have learned more about the neurophysiological changes resulting from chronic cocaine abuse, there has been an increasing effort to discover how specific medications may help to correct these alterations.

Our own research has identified a significant subgroup of chronic cocaine abusers who concurrently suffer from affective (mood) disorders: recurrent episodes of depression, or mood swings varying from highs to lows (bipolar disorder, formerly called manic-depressive illness). These studies, whose findings were replicated by Drs. Frank Gawin and Herbert Kleber at Yale University School of Medicine, suggest that medications that are typically used to treat mood disorders may be helpful in the subgroup of cocaine abusers with coexisting affective disorders. Indeed, in a recent study by Drs. Gawin and Kleber, a small group of cocaine abusers reported decreased craving and cocaine use after receiving the antidepressant drug desipramine, whether or not they had had a history of depression. Patients with manic-depressive illness were not given desipramine, since this medication may worsen such patients' mood disorders. Rather, they were treated with lithium carbonate, which is typically prescribed in such disorders. Again, the results were generally positive. Although the number of patients treated in this study was quite small, the findings suggest a potentially beneficial role for desipramine or lithium in the treatment of certain cocaine abusers. Although further research will be needed to reach more definitive conclusions about the effectiveness and safety of these or other medications in cocaine abusers, it is safe to say that a psychiatric evaluation can be extremely useful in helping to determine whether another potentially treatable disorder may be making a cocaine abuse problem worse.

Ann J., a 27-year-old laboratory technician, was hospitalized because of a three-year history of cocaine abuse. She stated that she had initially used cocaine at a party with a group of friends and had experienced a dramatic change in her mood. She said, "I never knew that I had been depressed until after I used cocaine. Then I finally knew what it was like to feel good." Unfortunately, the feelings of well-being caused by cocaine were short-lived, and she experienced steadily worsening mood swings as well as vocational, marital, and financial difficulties as a result of her cocaine abuse. She was hospitalized on the advice of her employer.

Ann was extremely depressed at her admission to the hospital and experienced some suicidal thoughts. Unlike most patients, however, Ann's depression did not improve at all during the course of her hospitalization. Although she participated in individual psychotherapy, numerous groups, and Narcotics Anonymous, she felt that she was "just going through the motions. I felt miserable and didn't really care if I got better." She complained of a poor appetite and weight loss while in the hospital, and she frequently awoke during the middle of the night and early in the morning. Since the latter symptoms are typically seen in nondrug users with affective (mood) disorders, and because we observed so little improvement in Ann's mood after several weeks of hospitalization, we treated her with the antidepressant drug desipramine at a dose of 150 milligrams a day. Within approximately two weeks, her mood gradually improved, she became much more hopeful, her sleeping and eating habits normalized, and her craving for cocaine diminished. She continued in individual psychotherapy and in Narcotics Anonymous and was able to use treatment much more to her advantage. She said, "My heart was in it now. I wanted to get better and I felt that I could."

Self-Help Groups: Alcoholics Anonymous, Narcotics Anonymous, Cocaine Anonymous. Alcoholics Anonymous (AA) and similar organizations, such as Narcotics Anonymous (NA) and Cocaine Anonymous (CA), are self-help groups whose aim is to help substance abusers achieve lasting sobriety. These world-wide organizations meet regularly so that members can share their recovery experiences and support each other in the strug-gle to avoid relapse. These programs support complete absti-nence from all drugs, including alcohol. Unlike the help of-fered by many professionals and social agencies, these groups are almost continuously available. Experienced group mem-bers (sponsors) help to care for newer members during peri-ods in which the risk of relapse is high. During the group meetings themselves, members hear others' stories of recovery and often find their first rays of hope in one of these meetings. The only requirement for membership is the honest desire to become drug and alcohol free. There are no fees or dues.

Rebecca D., a 30-year-old writer, was referred to Narcotics Anon-ymous by her family physician after she told him about her steadily increasing cocaine habit. Her reaction to her initial meeting was quite negative. "I entered a smoke-filled room and saw a bunch of tough-looking guys and sleazy-looking women, and I was convinced that none of these people had anything in common with me. Looking back on it, I know that I purposely sought out people who were different from me in order to give myself an excuse to not get involved and not give up cocaine.

"At that first meeting, though, I managed to meet one woman who had a lot on the ball and was very helpful. She encouraged me to come back to NA again and see if I liked it any better. I was pretty resistant, but I knew that my cocaine habit was pretty bad, so I decided to give it one more try. The second meeting seemed a little less dreary than the first. When I heard the speaker, I heard a lot of things that reminded me of myself, and my ears picked up a little bit when she started to talk about her recovery. I listened in on other people's conversations, and when I started to hear re-covery tales, I began to think, 'If these people can get straight, I can.' I went again, and some faces started to look familiar. People started getting more friendly, and I realized that there was a lot of warmth in NA, and people really care about each other. There is this mentality that we're all in this boat together, and that by helping out each other, we help ourselves.

"I struggled mightily with the first step of NA, which involved admitting that I was powerless over cocaine and other drugs and that my life had become unmanageable because of my addiction. When I finally accepted this step, though, I started to get better. I got myself a sponsor and I call her regularly. I have a list of phone numbers of other NA members, and I keep in regular contact with a group of people, just so that I don't drift into trouble without my knowing it. I've made some good friends in NA, and I've had to give up my old drinking and drugging companions. I honestly believe that going to that first meeting saved my life."

Outpatient Drug Programs. These programs, which may be affiliated with inpatient facilities, usually offer individual or group therapy, family counseling, and urine screening. Outpatient drug programs are frequently staffed by recovering drug addicts or alcoholics. Some outpatient cocaine programs have frequent group meetings (two to four times per week), require that their members attend a self-help group such as NA daily, and ask for urine screens two to three times per week. The intensity of these programs is designed to combat the powerful drug craving that many people experience when initially trying to stop cocaine.

Inpatient Treatment

Hospitalization. For some individuals with severe cocaine problems, a hospital may offer the safest place for treatment to begin. Hospitalization is usually indicated when outpatient treatment has failed, or when the patient's life circumstances make outpatient treatment either too risky or impossible. The following is a partial list of situations that would make us likely to recommend treatment in an inpatient facility.

Reasons for Hospitalization

Hospitalization is usually recommended if a cocaine abuser

1. Is actively threatening self-harm.
2. Is actively threatening to harm someone else.
3. Is taking such poor care of himself that he represents a significant threat to accidentally harm himself. This might include an individual who has recently begun to use drugs intravenously or someone who exposes himself to great physical danger in obtaining drugs.
4. Is dangerous to others and himself because of his recklessness and poor judgment, such as someone who regularly drives while intoxicated.

5. Has a poor system of social supports, such as an individual who lives with an active substance abuser.
6. Has severe medical or psychiatric complications as a result of cocaine abuse.
7. Is dependent upon alcohol or drugs other than cocaine and needs medical detoxification.
8. Is unwilling or unable to participate in an active outpatient treatment program.
9. Has failed in outpatient treatment.

Hospital treatment, which usually takes place on a specialized substance abuse unit, offers several major advantages over outpatient treatment. First, the hospital environment offers a safe refuge from cocaine at a time when addicts are least capable of resisting the drug on their own. The decreased availability of cocaine reduces drug craving (see Chapter 5) and offers patients enough time to learn that they can make a choice about their drug use. Another advantage of hospitalization is the fact that the patients immediately become part of a supportive peer group of other addicts who are similarly attempting to stop their drug use. Placement in a new, supportive environment offers addicts hope that they can overcome some of the loneliness and isolation that are so common among chronic drug abusers.

Family involvement is often a critical aspect of hospital treatment; relatives and friends of cocaine abusers are frequently angry, depressed, and desperately frustrated. They, too, need a great deal of support and education about the addictive process, its effects on family members, and ways in which they can rebuild their own lives (see Chapter 6 for further discussion about the effect of cocaine addiction on the family).

In addition to repairing strained relationships with loved ones, another task of hospitalization is the assessment of the patient's vocational or school situation (see Chapter 7). Since so many cocaine abusers eventually experience difficulty at work because of their drug use, vocational counseling is an important part of a drug rehabilitation program. Involvement of the employer in this process is sometimes quite helpful in improving work attendance and performance.

One important benefit of inpatient treatment is the fact that hospitalized patients can undergo medical, neurological, and psychiatric evaluation while they are drug-free. This is important in assessing and treating the common complaints of depression, anxiety, and insomnia, which are very difficult to evaluate in active cocaine abusers. It is initially virtually impossible to determine whether these symptoms are resulting from chronic cocaine use, from the withdrawal or "crash" that commonly follows the cessation of cocaine use, or from the numerous adverse events (such as loss of job, family, finances) that so frequently occur in the lives of cocaine addicts. Alternatively, these symptoms may have preceded the substance abuse and led to a misguided attempt at "self-medication" with cocaine or other drugs. In a drug-free hospital environment, we can begin to differentiate between the causes and effects of cocaine abuse and thus design a specific, individualized treatment program for each patient.

A final, critical advantage of hospitalization is its intensity: the doctors, nurses, social workers, and counselors working in an inpatient program have the opportunity to interact with patients 24 hours a day and can therefore observe their reactions to frustration, sadness, anxiety, anger, and happiness. Very often, subtle stresses that cause drug urges in cocaine abusers may not be readily observable in once- or twice-weekly psychotherapy. However, if a patient experiences the desire to use cocaine while he is in the hospital, he can talk about this feeling immediately. He may thus begin to understand more fully both the precipitants for his cocaine use and alternatives to giving in to his drug urges.

George F., a 36-year-old contractor, admitted himself to the hospital after his wife threatened to divorce him if he did not seek treatment for his cocaine abuse. George had used a variety of drugs since adolescence, with cocaine predominating during the past five years. He had financed his habit through heavy drug dealing; a threat to his family as the result of a recent transaction had led his wife to present him with an ultimatum.

When George first entered treatment, he was highly unmotivated, and he stated that the goal of complete abstinence was unrealistic. "I thought the staff were fools to think that we were supposed to stop using everything. I was looking to get my cocaine use under some control, and I was willing to consider stopping cocaine altogether. But the idea of stopping marijuana, which I had used every day for the last 15 years, was ridiculous. And I had never had an alcohol problem, so there was no way that I was about to stop drinking."

George received a great deal of confrontation from other patients and the treatment staff about his denial, and he was surprised and dismayed to find so little interest in his "war stories," which glorified his drug use and dealing. After he had been in the hospital for about 10 days, George's feelings began to change. "As all of these drugs were getting out of my system, I realized that I hadn't had one straight day in at least 15 years. I began to like the way I was feeling. I could think more clearly, and I started to get off on being straight. I started meeting people from NA that I really respected—guys who had been on the streets and who were learning a different way of life."

George's wife was concurrently learning more about addiction and enabling behavior (see Chapter 6). When George initially considered leaving the hospital prematurely, she received support from other relatives and the treatment staff for her insistence that he complete his treatment.

In individual psychotherapy, George began to understand how he used drugs and drug dealing in order to try to make up for feelings of low self-esteem. As he found other ways to feel good about himself, he began to feel less desperate about the prospect of a drug-free life. "Even when I left the hospital, I had tremendous reservations about the idea of staying straight. That's why I really held on to the NA slogan that tells you to take things one day at a time. One day didn't seem all that hard. The other saying that I held on to for a long time was, 'Fake it till you make it.' I faked it for a long time, but now, one year later, I really believe that my life is much better than when I was using drugs. I don't have thousands of dollars coming into my hand every few days, but I don't have all that money going out, either. My mind is clear, my business is good, and even my marriage has been salvaged. What helped me most about going into the hospital was having people on my back every day, constantly confronting me, and being in an environment where I couldn't just take off and get high whenever I wanted to. What I learned from that experience was that I could survive bad feelings, which is something that I hadn't forced myself to do for 20 years."

Therapeutic Communities. Therapeutic communities, sometimes known as "concept houses," are self-help residential treatment programs that are helpful in the rehabilitation of certain subgroups of chronic drug abusers, particularly those who have failed in other treatment modalities. These highly confrontational programs, which are usually run by former addicts, are based on a theory that drug addiction occurs because of a combination of immature personality traits and because of an environment that never compels the individual to face up to reality. A therapeutic community seeks to reverse this process by forcing its residents to face frustrations and uncomfortable feelings without seeking escape through drugs. It does so by creating a structured community that focuses on interpersonal concerns, particularly responsibility toward that community and the competent handling of aggression, hostility, and drug urges. Residents work their way up through the structured hierarchy of the community by demonstrating honesty and responsibility and by remaining drug-free. Those who do well in the system serve as role models for newcomers, and some graduates stay on to become staff members.

The highly confrontational nature of therapeutic communities, coupled with most addicts' ambivalence about seeking treatment, leads to a high dropout rate in these facilities. However, for those who stay in these programs, success rates on measures of drug abstinence and psychological maturity are relatively encouraging. Since therapeutic communities are stressful, psychologically difficult, long-term programs (they typically range from several months to two years in duration), they are usually not recommended as a first treatment effort. Rather, they are normally reserved for people who have failed at other treatment methods. The type of drug abuser who can benefit most from such a program tends to be someone with a chronic history of antisocial behavior or a longstanding record of poor vocational performance. For such individuals, the emphasis in therapeutic communities on honesty and responsibility can be quite beneficial.

Ed T., a 24-year-old cocaine abuser, was referred to a therapeutic community after he had failed in his second attempt at outpatient treatment following hospitalization. Ed had abused numerous drugs and alcohol since age 13, with intravenous cocaine abuse predominating during the past two years. He had financed his habit through drug dealing and street crime, and he had been arrested several times for drug-related offenses. He had dropped out of school at age 16 and had never worked for more than two consecutive months.

Ed entered a therapeutic community reluctantly, but he found it quite helpful. "When I was there, all distractions were taken away from me and I had to look at myself honestly for the first time. Everyone else in there was as good a con artist as I was, so all of my attempts to get over on people didn't fly. I used to take pride in being the best sneak thief in my town, but now I'm beginning to feel good about myself for being honest. I also think that I'm able to help other people with drug problems because I understand so well how addicts think." Ed was in a therapeutic community for one year. While there, he began working for his high school equivalency degree. When he obtained his degree, he joined the staff of the therapeutic community; he has been a highly respected employee there for the past year.

Halfway Houses. Halfway houses offer drug-dependent individuals the opportunity to live in a structured setting while getting involved in outpatient treatment and developing a lifestyle that does not revolve around drug use. Halfway houses are frequently helpful for people without solid living situations (such as people living with active substance abusers) who are about to be discharged from a drug treatment program. Since relapse rates for cocaine abusers tend to be highest in the period soon after discharge, a living situation supportive of abstinence is critical in helping the individual to establish important life-style changes during this difficult early period. Some halfway houses will accept people from the community who can benefit from an improved living situation, but who do not require a full hospital program.

How to Choose the Right Type of Treatment

Many people who have cocaine problems are unsure about how to help themselves. As we can see by the large variety of treatment methods listed above, choosing the proper form of treatment can be quite difficult. For a cocaine abuser who may already be ambivalent about stopping his drug use, the confusion created by the multitude of different treatment techniques can offer a further excuse to put off seeking help at all.

The best way for a cocaine abuser to choose a proper treatment program is to talk with someone who is knowledgeable about cocaine abuse. Some people with cocaine problems can benefit by speaking with their personal physicians, who may have some expertise in the area of cocaine abuse or can refer their patients to the proper individual or local agency for a consultation. People who do not have a personal physician can call a well-known hospital in their area to ask for a cocaine or drug abuse specialist. They can also call their state medical or psychiatric society, or a local medical school, and ask for the name of someone who specializes in the treatment of cocaine or other substance abuse. Alternatively, they may make an appointment at a reputable drug abuse treatment program in the area, or consult the list in Appendix B of this book in order to find a local drug abuse program. The national telephone helpline 1-800-COCAINE is another referral source for cocaine abuse programs. In the meantime, attending Narcotics Anonymous, Alcoholics Anonymous, or Cocaine Anonymous meetings may be helpful in initiating treatment. The numbers for these organizations can be found in any local telephone directory.

Seven General Rules for Cocaine Abusers Who Want to Quit

1. The time to stop using cocaine is now.

Procrastination is one of the most frequent tactics of drug abusers in their relentless avoidance of treatment. "I'll quit tomorrow" is a euphemism for "I have no intention of quitting today."

2. You should stop all at once, not gradually.

Gradually cutting down on cocaine is a fruitless venture. Each use of cocaine merely fuels the desire for more cocaine, and the recovery process is postponed indefinitely. Since cocaine withdrawal can cause depression, the drug should be stopped in a supportive setting.

3. Stop using all other drugs of abuse, including alcohol and marijuana.

This rule is frequently very difficult for cocaine abusers to accept. For many of them, alcohol and marijuana have never caused difficulties; they feel that they have a specific problem with cocaine, not with all drugs and alcohol. However, the use of alcohol or marijuana frequently represents an initial step toward relapse to cocaine. Since these drugs decrease inhibitions, one or two drinks may make a cocaine abuser feel somewhat less resolute about abstaining from cocaine than he felt while sober. This phenomenon is illustrated by the following case example:

Ralph M., a 33-year-old musician, was hospitalized because of cocaine abuse. He had been injecting cocaine intravenously every 15 minutes during the week prior to admission, causing serious abscesses on both arms. After being hospitalized for four weeks, he was discharged to home with the recommendation that he refrain from all drugs and alcohol. At first, he followed this regimen successfully, and he was able to refuse two offers to use cocaine during this period. However, approximately two months following his discharge, Ralph went out to dinner and ordered a half bottle of wine, to share with his wife. This had been his customary drinking pattern prior to his hospitalization; he drank only on weekends at restaurants, and he rarely imbibed more than two glasses of wine in an evening. That night, he saw a former cocaine-using companion at the restaurant. This friend, who had offered him cocaine several weeks previously, repeated the offer on this evening, and Ralph accepted. He later said, "I had had two glasses of wine, and I wasn't drunk at all; I was just feeling good. At the time that he offered me the cocaine, I truly believed that one line wouldn't hurt me. I know that I wouldn't have made that same decision, though, if I had been stone cold sober." Five days later, Ralph was again injecting cocaine every 15 minutes, and he was rehospitalized.

4. Change your life-style.

You cannot associate with drug-using companions, nor can you safely frequent establishments (bars, clubs) in which alcohol and drug use are central activities.

In Chapter 5, we discussed how craving increases during conditions that remind someone of his association with drugs. Thus, cocaine abusers frequently report urges for the drug when they associate with fellow users, when they enter areas in which they had previously used drugs, and when they see drug-related paraphernalia: mirrors, razor blades, straws, or needles. Since most follow-up studies of drug and alcohol abusers show that relapse is most common during the early stages of recovery, we advise people to avoid such stimuli diligently, especially early in their treatment. This leads us to our next rule.

5. *Whenever possible, avoid situations, people, places, etc. that cause drug urges.*

When it is impossible to avoid these situations, prepare yourself for them so that you will be able to handle them safely. Avoid testing yourself in order to monitor how well you are doing.

The phenomenon of testing oneself is quite common in drug users who are attempting to recover. They mistakenly believe that "passing a test" proves that their problem is well under control. A common assumption among those who challenge themselves is, "If I can survive this test, then I can get through anything, and I'll never use cocaine again." Unfortunately, nothing could be further from the truth. For example, a recovering cocaine abuser might test himself by walking past his dealer's house in order to convince himself that he does not need to go inside. Such behavior is likely to produce one of two unhappy results: he either fails the initial test by going inside the dealer's house, or he walks past the dealer's house and thereby becomes unafraid to do it again, thus becoming overconfident.

Overconfidence leads to a loss of the self-vigilance that is necessary for ongoing recovery. If a drug abuser does not fear his ability to relapse, he is at high risk to fail. One of the implications of the "one day at a time" concept so frequently espoused by Alcoholics Anonymous and similar groups is the fact that yesterday's abstinence does not ensure the same result today. Similarly, passing a test today does not mean that one will be able to resist drugs tomorrow. In fact, the resulting overconfidence from passing such a test may *decrease* the likelihood of remaining abstinent the next day. We therefore strongly advise people to avoid such tests.

6. *Find other rewards.*

Drug abusers frequently forget how to treat themselves well and enjoy themselves while drug-free. They often ignore hobbies, stop exercising, eat badly, lose touch with drug-free friends, lose interest in sex, ignore their physical well-being, and lead a life generally devoid of chemical-free pleasure. Learning how to reconnect with the drug-free world is one of the most difficult tasks for many cocaine abusers, some of whom have forgotten how to talk about anything except drugs. Self-help groups such as Narcotics Anonymous frequently hold social functions such as parties, dances, and sporting events in order to facilitate this process of reintegration. We also encourage our patients to reestablish relationships with old drug-free friends.

7. *Take good care of your body. Eat right and exercise.*

Researchers at Fair Oaks Hospital in Summit, New Jersey, have found that vitamin deficiencies are quite common in chronic cocaine abusers. This is not surprising, since cocaine is an appetite suppressant. The resumption of normal eating habits can therefore be an important part of the overall recovery process. Regular exercise is also potentially helpful for cocaine abusers, who often allow themselves to get into poor physical condition. Exercise can also be used as a social activity and as a substitute for cocaine use during periods of high drug craving. Finally, strenuous exercise may help to decrease anxiety in some individuals, perhaps through the release of opiate-like compounds in the brain called endorphins; the sense of well-being triggered by the release of these chemicals may decrease the desire for drugs.

Pathways to Recovery

There are many routes to recovery from cocaine abuse. Some individuals stop on their own, some go to self-help groups, some seek individual psychotherapy, others require hospitalization. Despite the variety of specific treatment methods, it does appear that certain general factors may facilitate recovery in patients who are dependent upon cocaine or other drugs of abuse:

1. Those individuals who have solid employment or school histories tend to fare better than those with erratic work

records. Remaining drug-free requires daily commitment
and follow-through, which must be accomplished regardless of one's mood. These characteristics are also necessary
in order to maintain a solid work record; those who are able
to wake up and go to work on days when they don't feel like
doing so are able to maintain better job histories than those
who give in to their desire to go back to bed.

2. Those people who will experience a definite, immediate
   adverse consequence as the result of further cocaine use
   tend to do well in treatment. Thus, the imminent fear of job
   loss, divorce, medical problems, or a jail term upon resumption of cocaine use can provide a powerful incentive
   for recovery. The success of such threats depends upon
   their credibility and the extent to which they will hurt the
   patient. This phenomenon is the theoretical basis for the
   "contingency contracting" treatment program that has
   achieved some success at the University of Colorado School
   of Medicine. Patients in this program who do not already
   have a clear negative consequence of further cocaine use
   help to design such a contingency themselves. Thus, a patient might write a letter to his employer, detailing his history of drug use and antisocial behavior. This letter is then
   held by the patient's therapist, who only mails it to the
   employer if the patient returns to drug use, as evidenced by
   positive urine screens.

3. Another factor that is particularly helpful in the recovery of
   some substance abusers is the ability to find a new source of
   hope and self-esteem. This may come from religious involvement, Alcoholics Anonymous or Narcotics Anonymous meetings, a helpful psychotherapy relationship, or a
   new love relationship uncontaminated by the difficulties
   brought about by the cocaine abuser's drug-related behavior.

Just as there are many pathways into cocaine abuse, there
are many routes out. Although abstinence from cocaine does
not guarantee happiness, a long-term study of abstinent alcoholics is encouraging: those alcoholics who had attained lasting sobriety functioned as well in most areas of their lives as
those who had never had a drinking problem.

9

Questions Frequently Asked About Cocaine

Questions Frequently Asked by the General Public

What is cocaine?

Cocaine is a stimulant drug derived from the South American coca plant, *Erythroxylon coca*. Its most important actions include stimulation of the central nervous system (the brain and spinal cord), and its ability to produce local anesthesia.

How much does cocaine cost?

Illicit ("street") cocaine costs approximately $50 to $100 a gram (1/28th of an ounce) in most metropolitan areas. Since buying in bulk lowers the price, an ounce of cocaine can be purchased for approximately $2000, which is still six times the current price of gold. Pharmaceutical (legal) cocaine, on the other hand, costs only about $50 an ounce (or about $1.79 per gram).

Is cocaine addicting?

For years, the generally accepted medical definition of addiction (dependence) required the presence of one or both of the following two factors: tolerance to the drug (the need for increased intake to obtain the same drug effect) and physical signs of withdrawal after stopping drug use. Since abruptly stopping cocaine use does not cause dramatic medical symptoms, cocaine was long considered to be physically nonaddicting. Although physicians were quick to point out cocaine's psychologically addicting qualities, many people using the drug or contemplating doing so saw this statement as a mere disclaimer. The World Health Organization has recently revised its definition of dependence, however. According to their new definition, drug dependence is "a state, psychic or also sometimes physical, resulting from the interaction between a living organism and a drug, and characterized by behavioral and other responses that always include a compulsive desire or need to use the drug on a continuous basis in order to experience its effects and/or avoid the discomfort of its absence." By this definition, which is similar to those of the National Institute on Drug Abuse and the American Psychiatric Association, cocaine is a highly addicting drug.

Is cocaine an aphrodisiac?

Cocaine has certainly developed a reputation as a sexual stimulant. In fact, one of cocaine's nicknames is the "love drug." For some people, cocaine does initially stimulate sexual drive and enhance sexual pleasure. However, in a survey of regular cocaine users, only 13 percent of respondents experienced sexual stimulation from cocaine. Moreover, as cocaine use becomes more chronic and habitual, interest in sex and ability to perform often decreases, as the user's interest in anything other than cocaine diminishes.

Questions Frequently Asked by Occasional Cocaine Users

Is it possible to overdose on cocaine?

Yes. Not long ago, deaths from cocaine overdose were quite rare. However, this tragedy is commonplace today. In 1985, 604 people were known to die as the result of cocaine overdose; the actual number of cocaine-related deaths is likely much higher. This represents an 1100 percent increase in the past decade. The major causes of death from cocaine overdose include 1) irregular heartbeat leading to cardiac arrest, 2) extremely high blood pressure that can cause bleeding into the brain (cerebral hemorrhage), 3) continuous epileptic seizures (status epilepticus), and 4) respiratory arrest.

Is it possible to overdose from snorting cocaine?

Yes. Many cocaine users incorrectly believe that snorting cocaine is "safe." Although freebase or crack smoking and intravenous cocaine use are medically more dangerous than intranasal use, snorting cocaine offers no guarantee against overdose. Overdoses are unpredictable; there is no single "lethal" dose of cocaine. Rather, each individual is vulnerable to overdose after a different amount of drug intake. A dose of cocaine that may barely affect one user may be fatal for another. Moreover, an overdose may occur during initial "experimentation" with the drug or after long-term use.

Another hazard of cocaine, regardless of the route of administration, is the fact that buying cocaine on the street is truly a blind purchase. You can never be sure exactly how much pure cocaine you are buying and how much adulterant ("cut") you are being sold. Therefore, if you are accustomed to buying highly adulterated cocaine and you are sold a batch of relatively pure cocaine, you may have a very serious reaction to the same amount of powder, which contains a much larger dose of cocaine.

I know that smoking freebase or crack or using intravenous cocaine can be very addicting, but is it possible to get addicted to cocaine just by snorting?

Yes. Most studies have shown that a significant percentage of the people being treated for chronic cocaine abuse are exclusively intranasal users. For example, 49 percent of the cocaine abusers admitted to our treatment unit and 61 percent of those calling the 1-800-COCAINE telephone helpline are exclusively intranasal users. Thus, "just" snorting offers no protection against cocaine-related problems.

An additional hazard of intranasal use is the risk of progression to other, more dangerous forms of cocaine abuse. Over 90 percent of intravenous users and freebase smokers began by snorting cocaine. Many of these people had previously assured themselves that they would never resort to these more hazardous forms of use. However, heavy cocaine use can alter previously solid judgment. Chronic users may become bolder and more careless, and they may take chances with their health that would previously have been unthinkable.

I am an occasional cocaine snorter, and I sometimes sell small amounts of cocaine to friends. How much legal trouble can I get into for this?

Possession of cocaine for any purpose other than legitimate medical use is illegal. Although cocaine possession is frequently classified as a misdemeanor, the sale of cocaine is generally considered a felony. Moreover, many states do not set a minimum amount of cocaine that needs to be sold in order to be considered drug trafficking. Enforcement of these laws varies from state to state and from judge to judge. Thus, the penalty for a first offense of cocaine possession may vary from a slap on the wrist to 20 years in prison. Penalties for the sale of cocaine may depend upon the amount sold. However, in some states, a first arrest for the sale of any amount of cocaine may be punishable by up to 99 years in prison.

Although I don't think I have a cocaine problem, I know that drug abusers are usually the last ones to know (or admit) that they have a problem. How would I know if I did have a cocaine problem?

If cocaine causes problems in your life, you have a cocaine problem. Thus, if the use of cocaine directly or indirectly leads to difficulties in your work, school, or relationships, or if it creates a financial strain, medical, psychological, or legal difficulties, then you have a cocaine problem. In addition, if your cocaine use has led you to behave in ways that you would have previously considered unacceptable, then you have a cocaine problem. A self-test for cocaine dependence can be found in Appendix A.

Even if you feel that your cocaine use is not currently a problem, there is still good reason to stop. Continued use is likely to result in increasingly difficult problems, along with the significant risk of developing cocaine dependence. The surest way to avoid these consequences is to stop all cocaine use while you feel that your use is controllable. If you do try to stop and find that you are not able to, we urge you to seek professional help.

I'm thinking of getting pregnant, and I like to snort cocaine. Should I give up the drug while I'm pregnant? How about while I'm nursing?

It is generally a good idea to avoid all drugs while you are pregnant. Recent evidence has underscored this point with regard to cocaine. Cocaine use during pregnancy has been associated with a higher incidence of miscarriages and premature separation of the placenta. In addition, babies born to women who used cocaine during pregnancy may be more tremulous and less interactive than normal infants.

As for nursing, small amounts of cocaine have been detected in the breast milk of nursing mothers. Thus, the use of cocaine by a woman who is breastfeeding directly exposes her baby to the toxic effects of the drug.

Can you get hepatitis just from snorting cocaine?

Yes. Hepatitis B and non-A, non-B hepatitis are transmitted via the blood and via intimate sexual contact. Although sharing needles provides the most frequent route of transmission from one person to another, sharing snorting paraphernalia may similarly spread the disease. A microscopic drop of blood from a straw, dollar bill, or "tooter" is sufficient to transmit the virus.

Can you get hepatitis more than once?

Yes. Although many people become immune after being exposed to hepatitis B, this does not confer immunity to non-A, non-B hepatitis, which can be contracted more than once. A relapse of hepatitis can also be precipitated by drinking alcohol, which has a direct toxic effect on the liver.

Can you get AIDS from using cocaine?

Yes. Intravenous drug abusers are one of the groups at highest risk of contracting AIDS, a deadly disease that attacks the immune system. The use of cocaine, as opposed to heroin or other drugs, neither increases nor decreases that risk.

I find that I don't enjoy cocaine as much as I used to. In fact, I get depressed and anxious on the drug. But I find myself using more in an attempt to reexperience the great highs that I used to get. What's wrong?

You are describing the typical symptoms of the transition from occasional cocaine use to compulsive use. If you do not stop, you appear to be headed for trouble. Initially, most occasional cocaine users experience euphoria from the drug. However, as continued use becomes more frequent and intensive, users tend to feel the opposite of euphoria; depression, anxiety, and irritability are common reactions. Many individuals respond as you did: they take more cocaine in an attempt to reexperience the euphoria. Unfortunately, the next stage in the progression of this pattern is generally characterized by paranoia, often accompanied by frightening hallucinations. The time for you to stop your cocaine use is now. If you cannot do it on your own, you should seek help immediately.

Questions Frequently Asked by People Dependent upon Cocaine

I know a lot of people who can snort one or two lines of cocaine and put it down. But, regardless of how much cocaine is around, I'll use it until it's gone. Why can some people use the drug with control while others can't?

There is no simple answer to this question. Many researchers are trying to determine what makes some people particularly vulnerable to cocaine addiction. Most experts believe that a combination of factors leads to addiction, including the user's response to cocaine, the availability of the drug, and life circumstances. For example, some research, including our own, has found an increased rate of mood disorders in chronic cocaine abusers. This has led to speculation that a history of depression or mood swings might increase one's risk for cocaine addiction. However, addiction cannot occur without drug availability, including a means to pay for the drug or a willingness to engage in illegal activities in order to do so.

It is important to keep in mind that no one starts out as a cocaine addict. Many people start out as "controlled users." However, some occasional users become addicts. Unfortunately, there is no way to predict ahead of time who will become dependent upon cocaine and who will not.

My cocaine use is out of control. I want to cut back to social use again. Any suggestions?

Once you have become dependent upon cocaine, the only way to regain control over your life is to stop all drug use completely. The path to cocaine addiction at some point becomes a one-way street, in which the route back to occasional use is blocked. Virtually everyone who enters treatment because of cocaine abuse has already tried to "cut back" dozens of times. Unfortunately, many of these individuals inflict a great deal of damage upon themselves and others before giving up on this approach. For you, the only two choices now are continued addiction or complete abstinence.

I was recently treated for cocaine abuse and was told that I not only have to give up cocaine, but all other drugs, including marijuana. They even want me to stop drinking. I've never had a problem with any other drugs, and I don't even like the taste of alcohol much. My only problem was with cocaine. Isn't the recommendation to give up other drugs and alcohol a little excessive?

Although many patients balk at our recommendation for complete abstinence from all drugs of abuse (including alcohol), we feel that this advice is sound. Using other drugs presents two risks for you. First, you may become dependent upon the other drug. For example, 60 percent of the cocaine abusers admitted to our unit use three or more drugs regularly, and nearly half are alcoholic. An aversion to the taste of alcohol unfortunately offers you no protection against the future development of alcoholism. A second hazard of alcohol or other drug use is the fact that even low doses of most drugs will decrease your inhibitions. Thus, even a relatively small amount of alcohol or marijuana may make you feel less committed to total abstinence from cocaine than you felt while completely sober. We have seen a large number of cocaine abusers return to cocaine use after having just one or two drinks. For a description of such a relapse, see page 137. Resolve, willpower, good judgment, and the best of intentions are all soluble in alcohol. If cocaine is available after you have had a couple of drinks, you may decide that "one line won't hurt," although you would know better while completely sober.

I am beginning to have trouble falling asleep after using cocaine, and I've been drinking more and using Valium to help me sleep. Should I worry about this?

Yes. Nearly half of the patients admitted to our treatment unit for cocaine abuse are also alcoholic, and about 15 percent have problems with sedative-hypnotic drugs such as Valium. The use of other drugs to mitigate the stimulant effects of cocaine or to buffer the symptoms of a cocaine "crash" is very common and quite dangerous. Unfortunately, the dependence upon alcohol or sedative-hypnotic drugs frequently continues even after the cocaine abuse has stopped.

I'm worried about my cocaine use. How do I go about finding help?

Admitting that you have a problem is an important first step. The types of treatment available for cocaine abuse vary in their approach, intensity, and cost. Chapter 8 of this book describes the various types of treatment methods that are available for cocaine abusers. If you are not sure which route to take, it would be helpful for you to consult someone in your area who is knowledgeable about cocaine abuse. That person will be best able to recommend a course of treatment for you. In order to find such a person, there are several paths you can take:

1. Ask your physician if he knows a knowledgeable person whom you can consult about the problem.

2. Call your state psychiatric or medical society and ask for the name of a person who specializes in drug dependence. Then try to make an appointment with that person.
3. Call a local medical school and ask for the name of the person who runs their drug abuse program or who teaches at the school about drug abuse. If that person cannot see you, he will be able to refer you to someone else knowledgeable in the field.
4. If you know of a good drug abuse program in your area, call the director and ask for a consultation or a referral. A nationwide list of treatment programs can be found in Appendix B.
5. If you do not know of a good drug abuse program in your area and none is listed in Appendix B, call the toll-free 1-800-COCAINE telephone helpline and ask for a referral to an appropriate person in your area.
6. In addition to one of the steps mentioned above, you can call your local chapter of Narcotics Anonymous, Cocaine Anonymous, or Alcoholics Anonymous and start attending their meetings.

Can psychotherapy help me to stop using cocaine?

There is no single form of treatment that will help every cocaine abuser. Psychotherapy, like all treatment approaches for cocaine abuse, is extremely valuable for some people and less effective in helping others to stop their cocaine use. Although abstinence is a common goal of virtually all forms of treatment, the approaches leading to this end point vary considerably. Some people benefit primarily from attending self-help groups such as Narcotics Anonymous, Cocaine Anonymous, or Alcoholics Anonymous. For others, certain medications may prove very useful. In some cases, hospitalization may be required in order to stop cocaine use. Conversely, there are cocaine addicts who have simply stopped on their own with no outside help. If you have questions about whether individual psychotherapy would be helpful for you, we suggest talking with someone who is knowledgeable about both drug abuse and psychotherapy. This person may be able to advise you about the treatment approach that is most likely to help you.

Does cocaine abuse run in families?

Since cocaine abuse has been common in this country only since the early 1970s, there is little information on the transmission of the problem from generation to generation. Since this type of research is carried out over decades, we will have to wait until the next century before we will have the answer to this question.

Questions Frequently Asked by Those Who Treat Cocaine Abusers

When do you recommend hospitalization for a cocaine abuser?

This is an area of some controversy. In general, the decision whether to hospitalize a patient is made on the basis of the severity of the problem.

There are several signs that would lead us to initially recommend hospitalization for a cocaine abuser: 1) suicidal or homicidal thoughts; 2) reckless behavior which indicates that the cocaine abuser is ignoring the consequences of his drug use; 3) addiction to another drug or alcohol; or 4) risk of imminent severe consequences of drug use, such as medical illness, job loss, arrest, or divorce. If a cocaine abuser does not meet any of the criteria mentioned above, and if he is willing and able to engage in an outpatient program, we may recommend outpatient treatment initially. For patients who are unsuccessful in outpatient treatment, hospitalization may be recommended as a backup plan.

I have read some very impressive statistics supporting certain treatments for cocaine abuse, such as desipramine and contingency contracting. Do you recommend using these methods for all cocaine abusers?

There is no single "best" treatment for all cocaine abusers. There are clearly some individuals for whom contingency contracting (see page 140 for further details) is extremely useful. However, there are other patients who will relapse despite such a contingency program and may then be worse off for having made such a contract. Thus, this form of treatment should only be offered after carefully evaluating the patient's total life circumstances and discussing the pros and cons of the treatment with the patient.

While some of the early work on the use of the antidepressant drug desipramine in cocaine abusers has been encouraging (see pages 127–128 for further details), the total number of patients who have been successfully treated with this medication is small. In addition, we have seen a number of people who have continued to use cocaine despite being given desipramine. Desipramine, like other forms of treatment, is not a panacea for cocaine abuse. However, it may be helpful for a certain segment of the cocaine-abusing population—particularly those individuals with coexisting mood disorders. Early research results are encouraging, but we emphasize the word "early." Much more evidence will be required before we can confidently prescribe desipramine or any other medication to certain subgroups of cocaine abusers.

Do you recommend urine screening for cocaine abusers who are in the hospital?

Absolutely. Since it is difficult for even experienced treatment personnel to detect cocaine use clinically, there is no substitute for urine screening as an instrument of detection and deterrence. In order for urine screening to be effective, however, the testing must be random, supervised, and accurate.

Do different laboratory techniques vary in their ability to detect cocaine in the urine accurately?

Yes. The best laboratory methodology for detecting cocaine use utilizes an enzyme immunoassay (EIA) technique such as EMIT, with confirmation of positive results by combined gas chromatography–mass spectrometry (GC–MS). Thin-layer chromatography (TLC), which is used in many laboratories, is less useful, because it can detect cocaine or its metabolite benzoylecgonine in urine for only about 12 to 24 hours after cocaine use.

How long does cocaine or its metabolites stay in the urine?

Enzyme immunoassay (EIA) techniques such as EMIT can detect cocaine or its metabolite benzoylecgonine for up to 48 hours after drug use. Combined gas chromatography–mass spectrometry (GC–MS) ordinarily can detect cocaine or benzoylecgonine in the urine for several days after drug use, although there have been rare reports of positive urine screens seven to eight days after cocaine use.

Questions Frequently Asked by Family Members of Cocaine Abusers

I have just found out that my son is addicted to cocaine. Did I do something wrong during his childhood that caused his drug problem?

This is one of the questions most commonly asked by parents of cocaine abusers. Frequently those who don't ask are reluctant to do so because they are afraid that they already know the answer. The answer, however, is not simple because there is no single "cause" of cocaine abuse. There is good evidence, for instance, that childhood trauma cannot be blamed as a cause of alcoholism. Although research on cocaine abuse is comparatively new, no studies have shown that specific childhood experiences or family interactions predispose an individual to the future development of cocaine abuse.

How can I tell if my teenage daughter is using cocaine?

If your daughter is using the drug frequently, you may notice a disturbance in her sleeping pattern, with late nights followed by daytime somnolence; she may be particularly moody and irritable; she may have frequent "cold" symptoms; she may lose weight rapidly; and she is likely to borrow (or steal) money from you frequently. She may develop problems in school, and she may leave the house for long periods of time without explanation.

These symptoms, in addition to an attitude of secretiveness and distrust, may be warning signs of cocaine use. However, it may be very difficult to detect cocaine use, particularly in its early stages. Therefore, it is important to keep the lines of communication open with your daughter and to have frank discussions with her about drugs.

My husband has just been hospitalized for cocaine abuse. What are the chances of his recovery?

Although cocaine addiction is a chronic illness with the potential for relapse always present, it is treatable. Although treatment outcome studies are in their preliminary stages, early results have been quite promising. Recovery from cocaine addiction, however, is a long-term process that involves hard work and sacrifices. It can be particularly difficult for family members when the recovering addict devotes a great deal of time and energy to treatment activities. Therefore, it is often helpful for family members of cocaine addicts to seek support of their own, such as individual therapy, Nar-Anon, or a similar support group.

I think my wife is addicted to cocaine. I have talked with her constantly about stopping, but it does no good. This drug is ruining our marriage, our kids, and our finances. But she keeps claiming that it's "no big deal." How can she keep saying this and what can I do?

You have provided a vivid illustration of why addiction is called a "disease of denial." It is this denial or minimization of the wreckage caused by drug abuse that makes living with an addict so painful and exasperating. It is your wife's illness of addiction that keeps her from seeing what cocaine is doing to her. She clearly needs treatment, and you may be able to help her get it. The best way to help her is to confront her with the consequences of her cocaine abuse in a clear, nonjudgmental, but firm manner. If your children are old enough to do so, you may involve them in the confrontation as well. The details of such an encounter, called an *intervention*, are described in Chapter 6. You must also think about what you will do if your wife does not accept treatment, for you must not allow yourself and the rest of your family to be destroyed by your wife's addiction. To obtain guidance and support during this process, we suggest that you speak with someone in a drug abuse treatment center who is experienced in performing family interventions. You might also find Nar-Anon meetings helpful, while your children may benefit from Alateen meetings if they are old enough. If your wife does enter treatment, we urge you to participate in the part of the program for family members, since the illness of addiction affects the entire family.

Appendix A

Self-Test for Cocaine Dependence

The following self-test consists of a list of questions designed to examine your use of cocaine and to identify the potential problems that the drug can cause. The questions are organized around the types of difficulties that are most frequently associated with cocaine use. Answer the questions honestly; there are no right or wrong answers. If you find yourself answering "yes" to even a few of the questions, you may have a significant cocaine problem, warranting serious attention. For advice on how to seek help, see Chapter 8 and Appendix B.

A. *Medical Problems*

1. Do you frequently have "cold" symptoms, nasal congestion, or nosebleeds?
2. Have you ever had a seizure (convulsion) as the result of cocaine use?
3. Have you ever had a frightening physical experience while on cocaine, such as severe heart palpitations or a feeling that you were in serious medical danger?
4. Have you ever used cocaine intravenously?
5. Have you ever used the same needle more than once?
6. Have you ever shared needles with other drug users?
7. Have you ever shared needles with other drug users that you suspected had hepatitis?

8. Have you ever shared needles with other drug users that you suspected had AIDS?
9. Have you ever had shortness of breath, difficulty breathing, or a serious cough as the result of freebase or crack smoking?

B. Psychological Problems

1. Do you continue using cocaine despite the fact that it makes you anxious? Jittery? Irritable? Restless? Belligerent?
2. Have you ever hallucinated while on cocaine?
3. Did the use of cocaine ever make you feel that there were people trying to harm you when in fact you know that they weren't?
4. Do you get depressed ("crash") when you stop using cocaine?
5. Do you use more cocaine in order to end the crash?
6. Do you use other drugs or alcohol in order to treat some of the undesirable effects of cocaine, such as insomnia, anxiety, depression, or restlessness?

C. Problems with Other People

1. Do other people complain about your cocaine use?
2. Do you find that you are choosing cocaine over the company of other people?
3. Do you use cocaine primarily when you are alone?
4. Has cocaine caused a lack of sexual interest?
5. Has cocaine impaired your ability to perform sexually?
6. Have you found yourself lying, cheating, manipulating, or stealing from friends or relatives because of your cocaine use?
7. Are you more irritable and curt around other people?
8. Have you found that an increasing number of your "friends" are drug-related acquaintances?
9. Have you ever lost an important relationship because of your cocaine use?
10. Do you find that more and more of your conversations are focusing on cocaine, to the exclusion of other topics that used to interest you?

D. Problems at Work or School

1. Do you get high at work or during school hours?
2. Has your work or school performance declined as your use of cocaine has increased?
3. Do you sometimes miss work or school either because you are high or because you are crashing?
4. Do you believe that you would be doing better at work or school if you did not use cocaine?

E. Financial Problems

1. Has your use of cocaine ever caused financial problems?
2. Have you ever spent money on cocaine that had been earmarked for something else?
3. Have you ever stolen money or anything else in order to pay for cocaine?
4. Have you ever "borrowed" money for cocaine and not paid it back?
5. Have you ever sold cocaine in order to finance your own drug use?
6. Has your income decreased because of poor business decisions made while intoxicated or in haste because you wanted to get high?
7. Have you ever lamented the amount of money you have spent on cocaine?

F. Legal Problems

1. Have you ever been arrested for cocaine use?
2. Have you ever driven a car while under the influence of cocaine?
3. Have you ever performed illegal acts in order to obtain cocaine?

G. Loss of Control

1. Have you ever told yourself that you would stop cocaine immediately, then changed your mind and pledged to stop the next day?
2. Do you find yourself constantly thinking about cocaine?
3. Do you dream about cocaine?

4. Do you get an urge to use cocaine when you are exposed to people, places, or things (such as mirrors or razor blades) that remind you of the drug?
5. Have you become extremely discouraged by your unsuccessful attempts to stop using cocaine?
6. Have you ever thought about suicide because of your fear that you will never be able to stop using cocaine?
7. Do you feel that you have lost a sense of right and wrong since you started using cocaine?
8. Do you find yourself justifying your behavior to yourself when you would have clearly seen this behavior as immoral or wrong before you started using cocaine?
9. Do you feel that you have to use cocaine if it is around?
10. Do you use whatever amount of cocaine is available—that is, do you use it until it is gone?
11. Do you use cocaine even after telling yourself that you won't?
12. Do you think you have a problem with cocaine?
13. Do you think that you are dependent upon cocaine?

Appendix B

Where to Find Help:
A State-by-State Guide to
Cocaine Abuse Treatment Facilities

Following is a nationwide list of cocaine abuse treatment facilities. For each facility, we have specified whether inpatient or outpatient services are offered. We recommend many of these programs based on our own personal knowledge of their reputations; we are grateful to Dr. Mark Gold and his colleagues at the 1-800-COCAINE telephone helpline for furnishing us with the names of recommended facilities in areas with which we are less familiar.

The treatment facilities listed below are not the only sources of help for cocaine abusers or their families; a more comprehensive description of treatment options and how to decide upon the proper form of treatment can be found in Chapter 8 and in Chapter 9.

State-by-State Guide to
Cocaine Abuse Treatment Facilities
(Please note that the listings below are all subject to change.)

ALABAMA

Hillcrest Hospital
6869 Fifth Avenue, South
Birmingham, AL 35212
    (205) 833-9000
    Inpatient

Charter Pines Recovery Center
251 Cox Street
Mobile, AL 36607
    (205) 432-8811
    Inpatient

ALASKA

Charter North Hospital
2530 DeBarr Road
P.O. Box 89019
Anchorage, AK 99508
  (907) 258-7575
  Inpatient and Outpatient

ARIZONA

Palo Verde Hospital
2695 Craycroft Road
Tucson, AZ 85717-0030
  (602) 795-4357
  Inpatient

Sedona Villa
P.O. Box 4245
West Sedona, AZ 86340
  (602) 282-3583
  (800) 874-9070 (in-state only)
  (800) 548-3008 (out-of-state)
  Inpatient

ARKANSAS

Charter Vista Hospital
Addictive Disease Unit
P.O. Box 1906
Fayetteville, AR 72702
  (501) 521-5731
  Inpatient

RESTORE
Riverview Medical Center
1310 Cantrell Road
Little Rock, AR 72201
  (501) 376-1200
  Inpatient

Addictive Disease Unit
Outpatient Clinic
2700 American Street
Springdale, AR 72764
  (501) 756-0412
  Outpatient

CALIFORNIA

Southwood Mental Health Center
950 Third Avenue
Chula Vista, CA 92011
  (619) 426-6310
  Inpatient and Outpatient

San Luis Rey Hospital
1015 Devonshire Drive
Encinitas, CA 92024
  (619) 753-1245
  Inpatient and Outpatient

Forest Farm
145 Camel Road
Forest Knolls, CA 94933
  (415) 488-9287
  Inpatient

Alvarado Parkway Institute
7050 Parkway Drive
LaMesa, CA 92041
  (619) 583-2111
  Inpatient and Outpatient

Dominguez Medical Center
New Beginnings
171 Bort Street
Long Beach, CA 90805
  (213) 639-2664
  Inpatient

New Beginnings
Century City Hospital
2070 Century Park East
Los Angeles, CA 90067
  (213) 277-4248
  Inpatient

Merritt Peralta Institute
Chemical Dependency Recovery
  Hospital
435 Hawthorne
Oakland, CA 94609
  (415) 652-7000
  Inpatient and Outpatient

Betty Ford Center at Eisenhower
39000 Bob Hope Drive
Rancho Mirage, CA 92270
  (619) 340-0033
  (800) 392-7540 (in-state only)
  (800) 854-9211 (out-of-state)
  Inpatient and Outpatient

Alcohol and Substance Abuse Unit
Mesa Vista Hospital
7850 Vista Hill Avenue
San Diego, CA 92123
  (619) 694-8300
  Inpatient and Outpatient

Haight-Ashbury Free Medical
  Clinic
529 Clayton Street
San Francisco, CA 94117
  (415) 621-2016
  Outpatient

COLORADO

Boulder Memorial Hospital
311 Mapleton Avenue
Boulder, CO 80302
  (303) 441-0526
  Inpatient and Outpatient

Cedar Springs Psychiatric
  Hospital
2135 Southgate Road
Colorado Springs, CO 80906
  (303) 633-4114
  Inpatient and Outpatient

CONNECTICUT

University of Connecticut
Health Center
263 Farmington Avenue
Farmington, CT 06032
  (203) 674-3423
  Inpatient and Outpatient

Silver Hill Foundation, Inc.
P.O. Box 1177
208 Valley Road
New Canaan, CT 06840
  (203) 966-3561
  Inpatient

Substance Abuse Treatment Unit
Connecticut Mental Health Center
34 Park Street
New Haven, CT 06519
  (203) 789-7282
  Outpatient

DELAWARE

Greenwood
1000 Old Lancaster Pike
Hockessin, DE 19707
  (302) 239-3410
  Inpatient

DISTRICT OF COLUMBIA

Psychiatric Institute of
  Washington
4460 MacArthur Boulevard, N.W.
Washington, DC 20037
  (202) 944-3400
  Inpatient and Outpatient

George Washington University
  Hospital
Burns Building, 10th Floor
2150 Pennsylvania Avenue, N.W.
Washington, DC 20037
  (202) 676-3355
  Outpatient

Department of Psychiatry
George Washington University
  Hospital
6th Floor, North
901 23rd Street, N.W.
Washington, DC 20037
  (202) 676-4078
  Inpatient

FLORIDA

Fair Oaks Hospital at Boca-Delray
5440 Linton Boulevard
Delray Beach, FL 33445
(305) 495-1000
Inpatient and Outpatient

Coral Ridge Hospital
4545 North Federal Highway
Fort Lauderdale, FL 33308
(305) 771-2711
Inpatient and Outpatient

Recovery Center
HCA Highland Park Hospital
1660 Northwest 7th Court
Miami, FL 33136
(305) 326-7008
Inpatient and Outpatient

Harbor View Hospital
1861 N.W. South River Drive
Miami, FL 33125
(305) 642-3555
Inpatient

GEORGIA

Psychiatric Institute of Atlanta
811 Juniper Street, N.E.
Atlanta, GA 30308
(404) 881-5800
Inpatient and Outpatient

Substance Abuse Unit
Charter Lake Hospital
P.O. Box 7067
Macon, GA 31209
(912) 474-6200
Inpatient

Ridgeview Institute
3995 South Cobb Drive
Smyrna, GA 30080
(404) 434-4567
Inpatient

HAWAII

Kahi Mohala
91-2301 Ft. Weaver Road
Ewa Beach, HI 96706
(808) 671-8511
Inpatient

Drug Addiction Services of
Hawaii
640 Kakoi Street
Honolulu, HI 96819
(808) 836-2330
Outpatient

Castle Alcoholism and Addiction
Program
Castle Medical Center
640 Ulukahiki Street
Kailua, HI 96734
(808) 263-4429
Inpatient and Outpatient

The Aloha House
P.O. Box 490
Paia
Maui, HI 96779
(808) 579-9584
Inpatient

The Blessing House
P.O. Box 703
Waipahu, HI 96797
(808) 671-3678
Inpatient and Outpatient

IDAHO

The Walker Center
P.O. Box 541
Gooding, ID 83330
(208) 934-8461
Inpatient

Substance Abuse Unit
Mercy Medical Center Care Unit
1512 12th Avenue Road
Nampa, ID 83651
    (208) 466-4531
    Inpatient

ILLINOIS

Chemical Dependence Program
Northwestern Memorial Institute
    of Psychiatry
320 East Huron
Chicago, IL 60611
    (312) 908-2255
    Inpatient and Outpatient

INDIANA

Chemical Dependency Unit
St. Vincent's Stress Center
8401 Harcourt Road
Indianapolis, IN 46280-0160
    (317) 875-4710
    Inpatient

Chemical Dependency Outpatient
    Unit
1717 West 86th Street
Indianapolis, IN 46260
    (317) 871-3810
    Outpatient

IOWA

Sedlacek Treatment Center
Mercy Hospital
701 Tenth Street, S.E.
Cedar Rapids, IA 52403
    (319) 398-6226
    Inpatient and Outpatient

KANSAS

C. F. Menninger Memorial
    Hospital
5800 West 6th Street
Topeka, KS 66606
    (913) 273-7500
    Inpatient and Outpatient

KENTUCKY

Our Lady of Peace Hospital
2020 Newburg Road
Louisville, KY 40232
    (502) 451-3330
    Inpatient and Outpatient

LOUISIANA

New Life Center
Depaul Hospital
1040 Calhoun Street
New Orleans, LA 70118
    (504) 899-8282
    Inpatient and Outpatient

Jo Ellen Smith Psychiatric
    Hospital
4601 Patterson Road
New Orleans, LA 70114
    (504) 363-7676
    Inpatient

Westbank Center for
    Psychotherapy
4601 Patterson Road
New Orleans, LA 70114
    (504) 367-0707
    Outpatient

MAINE

Mercy Hospital Alcohol Institute
116 State Street
Portland, ME 04101
    (207) 774-1566
    Inpatient and Outpatient

MARYLAND

Taylor Manor Hospital
College Avenue
Ellicott City, MD 21043
  (301) 465-3322
  Inpatient

MASSACHUSETTS

Alcohol and Drug Abuse
  Treatment Center
McLean Hospital
115 Mill Street
Belmont, MA 02178
  (617) 855-2781
  Inpatient and Outpatient

Addiction Treatment Unit
New England Memorial Hospital
5 Woodland Road
Stoneham, MA 02180
  (617) 665-1740
  Inpatient

MICHIGAN

Psychiatric Center of Michigan
35031-23 Mile Road
New Baltimore, MI 48047
  (313) 725-5777
  Inpatient and Outpatient

Harold E. Fox Center
900 Woodward Avenue
Pontiac, MI 48053
  (313) 858-3177
  Inpatient and Outpatient

Substance Abuse Unit
Henry Ford Hospital
Maple Grove Center
6773 West Maple Road
West Bloomfield, MI 48033
  (313) 661-6100
  Inpatient and Outpatient

MINNESOTA

Hazelden
15425 Pleasant Valley Road
Center City, MN 55012
  (612) 257-4010
  Inpatient and Outpatient

University of Minnesota Hospital
Box 393 Mayo
420 Delaware Street, S.E.
Minneapolis, MN 55455
  (612) 626-5651
  Inpatient and Outpatient

St. Mary's Rehabilitation Center
2512 South 7th Street
Minneapolis, MN 55454
  (612) 338-2229
  Inpatient and Outpatient

Alcohol and Drug Dependence
  Unit
Station 93
Rochester Methodist Hospital
201 West Center Street
Rochester, MN 55902
  (507) 286-7593
  Inpatient

MISSISSIPPI

Delta Medical Center
P.O. Box 5247
Greenville, MS 38704
  (601) 334-2200
  Inpatient

Riverside Hospital
P.O. Box 4297
Jackson, MS 39216
  (601) 939-9030
  (800) 962-2180 (in-state only)
  Inpatient

MISSOURI

The Edgewood Program
St. John's Mercy Medical Center
615 South New Ballas Road
St. Louis, MO 63141
  (314) 569-6500
  Inpatient and Outpatient

Alcohol and Chemical
  Dependency Unit
Jewish Hospital
216 South Kingshighway
St. Louis, MO 63110
  (314) 454-8570
  Inpatient and Outpatient

MONTANA

Rim Rock Foundation
1231 North 29th Street
Billings, MT 59107
  (406) 248-3175
  Inpatient

Alcohol and Drug Program
St. James Hospital East
2500 Continental Drive
Butte, MT 59701
  (406) 723-4341
  Inpatient

NEBRASKA

Alcohol Treatment Center
Immanuel Medical Center
6901 North 72nd
Omaha, NE 68122
  (402) 572-2016
  Inpatient and Outpatient

NEVADA

Care Unit
Community Hospital of
  North Las Vegas
1409 East Lake Meade Boulevard
North Las Vegas, NV 89030
  (702) 642-6905
  Inpatient

Truckee Meadows Hospital North
2100 El Rancho Drive
Sparks, NV 89431
  (702) 323-0478
  Inpatient and Outpatient

NEW HAMPSHIRE

Hampstead Hospital
East Road
Hampstead, NH 03841
  (603) 329-5311
  Inpatient

Substance Abuse Unit
Nashua Brookside Hospital
11 Northwest Boulevard
Nashua, NH 03063
  (603) 886-5000
  Inpatient and Outpatient

Spofford Hall
Box 225
Spofford, NH 03462
  (603) 363-4545
  (800) 451-1716 (out-of-state)
  Inpatient

NEW JERSEY

Fair Oaks Hospital
1 Prospect Street
Summit, NJ 07901
  (201) 522-7000
  Inpatient and Outpatient

NEW MEXICO

Vista Sandia Hospital
501 Alameda Avenue, N.E.
Albuquerque, NM 87113
  (505) 823-2000
  Inpatient

NEW YORK

Stony Lodge Hospital, Inc.
P.O. Box 1250
Briarcliff Manor, NY 10510
  (914) 941-7400
  Inpatient and Outpatient

Bry Lin Hospital, Inc.
Rush Hall Chemical Dependency
  Treatment Program
1263 Delaware Avenue
Buffalo, NY 14209
  (716) 886-8200
  Inpatient and Outpatient

Falkirk Psychiatric Hospital
P.O. Box 194
Central Valley, NY 10917
  (914) 928-2256
  Inpatient

Regent Hospital
425 East 61st Street
New York, NY 10021
  (212) 935-3400
  Inpatient and Outpatient

NORTH CAROLINA

Appalachian Hall
P.O. Box 5534
Asheville, NC 28813
  (704) 253-3681
  Inpatient and Outpatient

Highland Hospital
49 Zillicoa Street
P.O. Box 1101
Asheville, NC 28802
  (704) 254-3201
  Inpatient and Outpatient

NORTH DAKOTA

Hartview Foundation
1406 N.W. 2nd Street
Mandan, ND 58554
  (701) 663-2321
  Inpatient and Outpatient

OHIO

Emerson A. North Hospital
5642 Hamilton Avenue
Cincinnati, OH 45224
  (513) 541-0135
  Inpatient

Woodruff Hospital
1950 East 89th Street
Cleveland, OH 44106
  (216) 795-3700
  Inpatient

OKLAHOMA

Chemical Dependency Unit
Presbyterian Hospital
707 N.W. 6th Street
Oklahoma City, OK 73102
  (405) 232-0777
  Inpatient

Presbyterian Hospital
1100 Classen Drive
Oklahoma City, OK 73103
  (405) 235-8364
  Outpatient

Shadow Mountain Institute
6262 South Sheridan Road
Tulsa, OK 74133
  (918) 492-8200
  Inpatient

OREGON

Wilshire Psychiatric Group
10490 S.W. Eastridge Street
Portland, OR 97225
  (503) 292-9101
  Inpatient and Outpatient

PENNSYLVANIA

The Fairmount Institute
561 Fairthorne Street
Philadelphia, PA 19128
  (215) 487-4102
  Inpatient

St. Francis Medical Center
Chemical Dependency Program
45th and Penn Avenues
Pittsburgh, PA 15201
  (412) 622-4580/4511
  Inpatient and Outpatient

RHODE ISLAND

Butler Hospital
345 Blackstone Boulevard
Providence, RI 02906
  (401) 456-3700
  Inpatient

SOUTH CAROLINA

Fenwick Hall Hospital
P.O. Box 688
1709 River Road
Johns Island, SC 29455
  (803) 559-2461
  Inpatient

SOUTH DAKOTA

River Park Inc.
P.O. Box 1216
Pierre, SD 57501
  (605) 224-6177
  Inpatient

TENNESSEE

Peninsula Psychiatric Hospital
Rt. 2, Box 233
Louisville, TN 37777
  (615) 970-9800
  Inpatient and Outpatient

Addictive Disease Unit
Lakeside Hospital
2911 Brunswick Road
Memphis, TN 38134
  (901) 377-4700
  Inpatient and Outpatient

TEXAS

Brookhaven Psychiatric Pavilion
7 Medical Parkway
Dallas, TX 75234
  (214) 247-1000
  Inpatient and Outpatient

Substance Abuse Program
Timberlawn Psychiatric
  Hospital, Inc.
4600 Samuels Boulevard
P.O. Box 11288
Dallas, TX 75223
  (214) 381-7181
  Inpatient and Outpatient

UTAH

St. Benedict's ACT Center
1255 East 3900 South
Salt Lake City, UT 84124
  (801) 263-1300
  Inpatient and Outpatient

VERMONT

Brattleboro Retreat
75 Linden Street
Brattleboro, VT 05301
  (800) 451-4203
  (802) 257-7785
  Inpatient and Outpatient

Champlain Drug and Alcohol
  Services
45 Clark Street
Burlington, VT 05401
  (802) 863-3456
  Outpatient

VIRGINIA

Chemical Dependency Treatment
  Program
David C. Wilson Hospital
2101 Arlington Boulevard
Charlottesville, VA 22903
  (804) 977-1120
  Inpatient

New Beginnings at Serenity
  Lodge
2097 South Military Highway
Chesapeake, VA 23320
  (804) 543-6888
  Inpatient

Psychiatric Institute of Richmond,
  Inc.
3001 Fifth Avenue
Richmond, VA 23222
  (804) 329-4392
  Inpatient

WASHINGTON

Kirkland Care Unit Hospital
10322 N.E. 132nd Street
Kirkland, WA 98033
  (206) 821-1122
  Inpatient

WEST VIRGINIA

Highland Hospital
300 56th Street
P.O. Box 4359
Charleston, WV 25364
  (304) 925-4756
  Inpatient and Outpatient

WISCONSIN

RiverWood Center
445 Court Street North
Prescott, WI 54021
  (715) 262-3286
  Inpatient and Outpatient

Milwaukee Psychiatric Hospital
1220 Dewey Avenue
Wauwatosa, WI 53213
  (414) 258-4094
  Inpatient and Outpatient

WYOMING

Substance Abuse Unit
Wyoming State Hospital
P.O. Box 177
Evanston, WY 82930
  (307) 789-3464
  Inpatient

Appendix C

Bibliography

Aigner TG, Balster RL: Choice behavior in rhesus monkeys: cocaine versus food. Science 201:534–535, 1978

Alcoholics Anonymous. New York, AA World Services, 1976

Anker AL, Crowley TJ: Use of contingency contracts in specialty clinics for cocaine abuse, in Problems of Drug Dependence 1981 [Research Monograph 41]. Edited by Harris LS. Rockville, Md, National Institute on Drug Abuse, 1982

Ashley R: Cocaine: Its History, Uses, and Effects. New York, St. Martin's Press, 1975

Benchimol A, Bartoll H, Desser KB: Accelerated ventricular rhythm and cocaine abuse. Annals of Internal Medicine 88:519–520, 1978

Byck R: Cocaine Papers: Sigmund Freud. New York, Stonehill Publishing Company, 1974

Caffrey RJ: Counter-attack on cocaine trafficking: the strategy of drug law enforcement. Bulletin on Narcotics 36:57–63, 1984

Chasnoff IJ, Burns WJ, Schnoll SH, et al: Cocaine use in pregnancy. New England Journal of Medicine 313:666–669, 1985

Coca paste and freebase—new fashions in cocaine use. Drug Abuse and Alcoholism Newsletter 9(3), 1980

Cohen S: Recent developments in the abuse of cocaine. Bulletin on Narcotics 36:3–14, 1984

Conway JP: Significant others need help, too. Alcoholism treatment is just as important to the rest of the family. Focus on Alcohol and Drug Issues 4:17–19, 1981

Dackis CA, Gold MS: New concepts in cocaine addiction: the dopamine depletion hypothesis. Neuroscience and Biobehavioral Reviews 9:469–477, 1985

DuPont RL Jr: Getting Tough on Gateway Drugs: A Guide for the Family. Washington, DC, American Psychiatric Press, 1984

Ellinwood EH, Kilbey MH: Cocaine and Other Stimulants. New York, Plenum Press, 1977

Estroff TW, Gold MS: Medical and psychiatric complications of cocaine abuse with possible points of pharmacological treatment, in Advances in Alcohol and Substance Abuse. Edited by Stimmel B. New York, Haworth Press, 1986

The evil empire. Newsweek, February 25, 1985, pp 14–18

Fischman MW, Schuster CR, Resnekov I, et al: Cardiovascular and subjective effects of intravenous cocaine administration in humans. Archives of General Psychiatry 33:983–989, 1976

Gawin FH, Kleber HD: Abstinence symptomatology and psychiatric diagnosis in cocaine abusers. Archives of General Psychiatry 43:107–113, 1986

Gawin FH, Kleber HD: Cocaine abuse treatment: open pilot trial with desipramine and lithium carbonate. Archives of General Psychiatry 41:903–909, 1984

Gay GR: The deadly delights of cocaine. Emergency Medicine 2:67–81, 1983

Gold MS: 800-COCAINE. New York, Bantam Books, 1984

Gold MS, Verebey K: The psychopharmacology of cocaine. Psychiatric Annals 14:714–723, 1984

Grabowski J: Cocaine: Pharmacology, Effects, and Treatment of Abuse [Research Monograph 50]. Rockville, Md, National Institute on Drug Abuse, 1984

Helfrich AA, Crowley TJ, Atkinson CA, et al: A clinical profile of 136 cocaine abusers, in Problems of Drug Dependence 1982 [Research Monograph 43]. Edited by Harris LS. Rockville, Md, National Institute on Drug Abuse, 1983

Itkonen J, Schnoll S, Glassroth J: Pulmonary dysfunction in "freebase" cocaine users. Archives of Internal Medicine 144:2195–2197, 1984

Javaid JI, Fischman MW, Schuster CR, et al: Cocaine plasma concentration: relation to physiological and subjective effects in humans. Science 202:227–228, 1978

Jeri FR, Sanchez C, Del Dozo T: The syndrome of coca paste: observations in a group of patients in the Lima area. Journal of Psychoactive Drugs 10:361–370, 1978

Jones RT: Marihuana-induced "high": influence of expectations, setting and previous drug experience. Pharmacological Review 23:359–369, 1971

Kellermann JL: A Guide for the Family of the Alcoholic. New York, Al-Anon Family Group Headquarters

Khantzian EJ: Extreme case of cocaine dependence and marked improvement with methylphenidate treatment. American Journal of Psychiatry 140:784–785, 1983

Khantzian EJ: The self-medication hypothesis of addictive disorders: focus on heroin and cocaine dependence. American Journal of Psychiatry 142:1259–1264, 1985

Kids and cocaine. Newsweek, March 17, 1986, pp 58–65

Kozel NJ, Adams EH: Cocaine Use in America: Epidemiologic and Clinical Perspectives [Research Monograph 61]. Rockville, Md, National Institute on Drug Abuse, 1985

Mule SJ: Cocaine: Chemical, Biological, Social, and Treatment Aspects. Cleveland, CRC Press, 1977

Narcotics Anonymous. Van Nuys, Calif, NA World Office, 1982

National Directory of Drug Abuse and Alcoholism Treatment and Prevention Programs. Rockville, Md, National Institute on Drug Abuse and National Institute on Alcohol Abuse and Alcoholism, 1985

National Institute on Drug Abuse: National Household Survey on Drug Abuse. Rockville, Md, National Clearinghouse for Drug Abuse Information, 1982

Nelson C: Styles of Enabling in the Codependents of Cocaine Abusers. San Diego, United States International University, 1984

Pearman K: Cocaine: a review. Journal of Laryngology and Otology 93:1191–1199, 1979

Perez-Reyes M, DiGuiseppi S, Ondrusek G, et al: Freebase cocaine smoking. Clinical Pharmacology and Therapeutics 32:459–465, 1982

Peterson RC, Stillman RC: Cocaine [Research Monograph 13]. Rockville, Md, National Institute on Drug Abuse, 1977

Post RM: Cocaine psychoses: a continuum model. American Journal of Psychiatry 132:225–231, 1975

Post RM, Kotin J, Goodwin FR: The effects of cocaine on depressed patients. American Journal of Psychiatry 131:511–517, 1974

Resnick RB, Kestenbaum RS, Schwartz LK: Acute systemic effects of cocaine in man: a controlled study by intranasal and intravenous routes. Science 195:696–698, 1977

Rounsaville BJ, Gawin F, Kleber H: Interpersonal psychotherapy adapted for ambulatory cocaine abusers. American Journal of Drug and Alcohol Abuse 11:171–191, 1985

Schnoll SH, Daghestani AN, Hansen TR: Cocaine dependence. Resident and Staff Physician 30:24–31, 1984

Schuckit M: Subjective responses to alcohol in sons of alcoholics and control subjects. Archives of General Psychiatry 41:879–884, 1984

Schulamith L, Straussner A, Weinstein DL, et al: Effects of

alcoholism on the family system. Health and Social Work 4:111–127, 1979

Siegel RK: Cocaine hallucinations. American Journal of Psychiatry 135:309–314, 1978

Siegel RK: Cocaine smoking disorders: diagnosis and treatment. Psychiatric Annals 14:728–732, 1984

Smith DE, Wesson DR: Cocaine. Journal of Psychedelic Drugs 10:351–360, 1978

Smith DE, Wesson DR: Treating the cocaine abuser. Center City, Minn, Hazelden Foundation, 1985

Stephen M, Prentice R: Developing an Occupational Drug Abuse Program. Rockville, Md, National Institute on Drug Abuse, 1978

Taylor D, Ho BT: Neurochemical effects of cocaine following acute and repeated injection. Journal of Neuroscience Research 3:95–101, 1977

Twelve Steps and Twelve Traditions. New York, AA World Services, 1980

Vaillant GE: The Natural History of Alcoholism: Causes, Patterns, and Paths to Recovery. Cambridge, Mass, Harvard University Press, 1983

Van Dyke C, Barash PG, Jatlow P, et al: Cocaine: plasma concentrations after intranasal applications in man. Science 191:859, 1976

Van Dyke C, Byck R: Cocaine. Scientific American 246:128–141, 1982

Walsh JM, Hawks RL: Employee Drug Screening. Rockville, Md, National Institute on Drug Abuse, 1986

Washton AM, Gold MS: Chronic cocaine abuse: evidence for adverse effects on health and functioning. Psychiatric Annals 14:733–743, 1984

Weiss RD, Goldenheim PD, Mirin SM, et al: Pulmonary dysfunction in cocaine smokers. American Journal of Psychiatry 138:1110–1112, 1981

Weiss RD, Mirin SM: Drug, host and environmental factors in the development of chronic cocaine abuse, in Substance Abuse and Psychopathology. Edited by Mirin SM. Washington, DC, American Psychiatric Press, 1984

Weiss RD, Mirin SM, Michael JL, et al: Psychopathology in chronic cocaine abusers. American Journal of Drug and Alcohol Abuse 12:17–29, 1986

Weiss RD, Pope HG Jr, Mirin SM: Treatment of chronic cocaine abuse and attention deficit disorder, residual type, with magnesium pemoline. Drug and Alcohol Dependence 15:69–72, 1985

Welti CV, Wright RK: Death caused by recreational cocaine use. Journal of the American Medical Association 241:2519–2522, 1979

Zinberg NE: Social interactions, drug use, and drug research, in Substance Abuse: Clinical Problems and Perspectives. Edited by Lowinson JH, Ruiz P. Baltimore, Williams and Wilkins, 1981

Index

Accidents, 38–40
Acquired Immune Deficiency
    Syndrome. *See* AIDS
Addiction (case study), 85–89. *See
    also* Cocaine abuse treatment;
    Cocaine dependence;
    Cocaine intoxication
"Addictive personality" theory,
    57–58
Adulterants ("Cuts"), 10, 24,
    37–38
AIDS (Acquired Immune
    Deficiency Syndrome), 36, 146
Amphetamine, 7–8
Anger, families', 93
Aphrodisiac, cocaine as, 31, 142
Availability, 2–3

Behavior
    effects of long-term cocaine use
        on, 49–53
    stereotyped, 47–48
    See also Cocaine dependence
Biological factors. *See* Cocaine
    dependence
Biological markers, 63–64
Brain function
    adverse reactions, 53–54
    behavioral effects of long-term
        cocaine use on, 49–53

effects of cocaine on, 45–49
elements of, 41–45
Burns, 37
Business
    effects of cocaine on, 114–116
    See also Workplace and
        cocaine

Case studies, 80–90
Classical conditioning, 70–72
Coca Cola, 6
Cocaine abuse treatment
    choosing the right type,
        135–136
    entering treatment, 122–124
    finding help, 148–149
    inpatient methods, 130–135
    outpatient methods, 124–130
    pathways to recovery, 139–140
    questions about, 150–151
    rules for quitting, 136–139
    See also Cocaine dependence
Cocaine dependence
    behavioral factors, 69–72
    biological factors, 60–64
    case studies, 80–89
    course and development of,
        73–80
    psychological factors, 57–60
    social factors, 64–69

175

Cocaine dependence
(continued)
   World Health Organization
      views on, 55–56
Cocaine epidemic
   history of use, 4–8
   international trade, 10–11
   manufacture and distribution,
      8–10
   scope of problem, 1–3
Cocaine intoxication, 14
Cocaine trade, international,
   10–11
Coca leaves, 4, 8–9
Coca paste, 17–18
Co-dependent, 100
"Concept houses." *See*
   Therapeutic communities
Conditioned stimuli. *See* Classical
   conditioning
Consciousness and arousal, 45
"Contingency contracting," 140,
   150
Convulsions. *See* Seizures
Cost. *See* Price
Costs to business. *See* Business
"Crack," 3. *See also* Freebase
Craving, 71–72
Cultural factors. *See*
   Sociocultural factors
"Cuts." *See* Adulterants

Death from cocaine use, 27–28,
   38–40
Definition, 4, 141
Denial, 75–80, 95–96
Dependence. *See* Cocaine
   dependence
Depression, 49–50
Detection, 151–152. *See also*
   Business
Dopamine. *See* Brain function
Drug dependence syndrome,
   73–77
Drug paraphernalia, 32–37

EAPs. *See* Employee Assistance
   Programs
Effects of cocaine on the body
   adulterants used, 24
   breakdown within the body,
      23–24

death from use, 27–28
   medical complications, 25–26,
      29–40
   physical effects, 24–25
   pseudocholinesterase, 23–24
   overdose, 27
Employee Assistance Programs
   (EAPs), 116–119
Enabling, 96–101
Endocarditis, 36–37
Endorphins, 64
Erythroxyline, 5
Experimentation (case study),
   81–82

Familial factors, 66–67
Families of cocaine abusers
   avoidance mechanisms, 95–101
   events common to, 92–93
   how relatives can help, 101–103
   questions asked by, 152–154
   recovery, 103–105
   responses to the abuser, 93–95
Family studies of alcoholism,
   61–63
Fear, families', 94
Federal Harrison Narcotics Act of
   1914. *See* Harrison Narcotics
   Act of 1914
Folklore, 4
Freebase, 3, 18–20
Freud, Sigmund, 5

Genetics, role of in alcoholism,
   61–62
Guilt, family, 93

Harrison Narcotics Act of 1914,
   6–7, 67
Heart valve, infection of. *See*
   Endocarditis
Hepatitis, 33–36, 145–146
History of cocaine use
   folklore, 4
   Freud, Sigmund, 5
   Mariani, Angelo, 5–6
   medicinal use, 4
Homicide, 39–40
Hospitalization, 130–133, 150

Importation. *See* Cocaine trade,
   international

Intervention, 101–103
Intranasal use, 13–16, 29–30, 143–144
Intravenous use, 21–22, 32–37

Kindling phenomenon, 48–49

Laboratory techniques, 151–152
Law enforcement, 10–11. *See also* Legislation
Laws. *See* Legislation.
Legislation, 7, 144
Literature, cocaine in, 6
Lung problems, 30, 37–38

Manufacture of cocaine, 8–10
MAO. *See* Monoamine oxidase
Mariani, Angelo, 5–6
Media, role of, 7
Medical complications from cocaine. *See* Effects of cocaine on the body
Medication used in treatment of abuse, 127–128
Mental illness, 53–54. *See also* Psychiatric symptoms
Monoamine oxidase, 63–64

Needles. *See* Drug paraphernalia
Nerve cell. *See* Brain function
Neurotransmitter. *See* Brain function
Norepinephrine. *See* Brain function
Nose problems, 29–30

Occasional use (case study), 81–82
"On Coca," 5
Operant reinforcement, 70
Outpatient drug programs, 130
Overdose, 27–28, 142–143

Paraphernalia. *See* Drug paraphernalia
Pavlov, Ivan. *See* Classical conditioning
Physiological effects, 14–17
See also Effects of cocaine on the body
Pleasure, perception of, 45–47
Pregnancy, 32, 145

Price, 2, 9–10, 18, 141
Problem use (case study), 83–85
Pseudocholinesterase, 23–24
Psychiatric symptoms, medical complications due to, 38–40
Psychological factors in cocaine dependence. *See* Cocaine dependence
Psychosis, cocaine, 50–53
Psychotherapy, 125–127, 149

Questions asked about cocaine
by cocaine addicts, 146–150
by family members, 152–154
by general public, 141–142
by occasional users, 142–146
by those who treat abusers, 150–152

Recovery, pathways to, 139–140
Recovery for families of abusers, 103–105
Regular use (case study), 82–83
Relatives, 101–103
Religious factors in drug use, 69
Risk factors, 53–54, 62–63

Scope of problem, 1–3
Seizures, 31, 47–48
Self-help groups, 128–130
"Self-medication" theory, 58–59
Sexual difficulties, 31
Shame, families', 94
Skin infections, 32–33
Smoking cocaine, 16–20, 30
Smuggling. *See* Cocaine trade, international
"Snorting." *See* Intranasal use
Social factors, 65–66, 68–69
Sociocultural factors, 67–69
"Speedballing," 3, 22. *See also* Intravenous use
State-dependent learning, 59–60
Suicide, 38

Teenagers, symptoms of use in, 152
Therapeutic communities, 133–135
Treatment. *See* Cocaine abuse treatment
Trends in American drug use, 6–8

Vietnam War, drug use during, 68–69

Viral hepatitis. *See* Hepatitis

Vitamin deficiencies, 30–31

Urine screening, 115–116

Uses of cocaine. *See* Intranasal use; Intravenous use; Smoking cocaine

WHO. *See* World Health Organization.

Work performance, 111. *See also* Workplace and cocaine

Workplace and cocaine
  hazards, 109–111
  reasons for use, 108–109
  response of business, 114–119
  use by executives, 111–114

World Health Organization, views on drug dependence, 55–56